SCHIZOPHRENIA

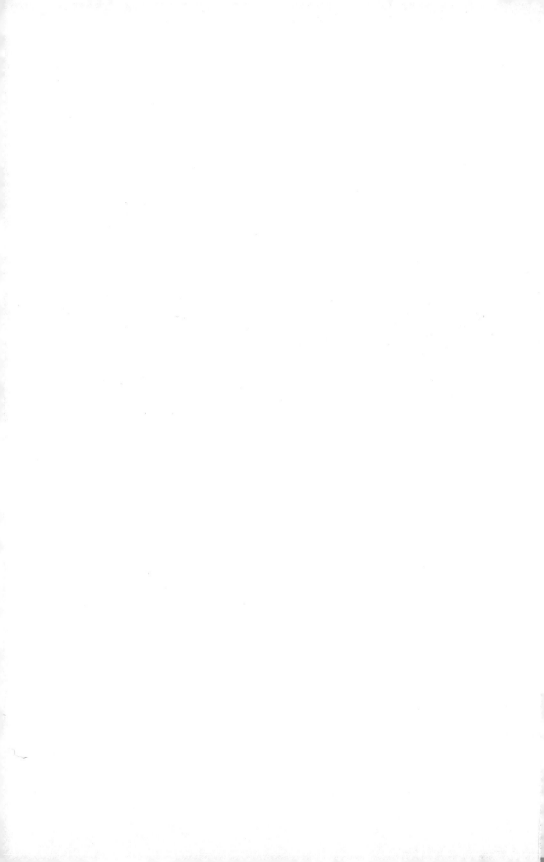

SCHIZOPHRENIA

Science, Psychoanalysis, and Culture

Kevin Volkan and Vamık Volkan

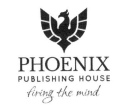

PHOENIX
PUBLISHING HOUSE
firing the mind

First published in 2022 by
Phoenix Publishing House Ltd
62 Bucknell Road
Bicester
Oxfordshire OX26 2DS

British Library Cataloguing in Publication Data

A C.I.P. for this book is available from the British Library

ISBN-13: 978-1-912691-94-4

Typeset by vPrompt eServices Pvt Ltd, India

Printed in the United Kingdom

www.firingthemind.com

Contents

About the authors ix

About this book xiii

Part I
Schizophrenia: Epidemiology, causes, neurobiology,
pathophysiology

1. Introduction and overview of schizophrenia 3

2. Causes of schizophrenia 8

3. Neurobiology of schizophrenia 30

4. Brain structure and schizophrenia 34

5. Cognition and schizophrenia 37

6. Social-cognitive and emotional recognition impairment
   in schizophrenia 40

7. Treatment of schizophrenia 43

8. Non-psychodynamic therapeutic approaches to treating
   schizophrenia 57

9. Recovery from schizophrenia   60

10. Prevention of schizophrenia   62

Part II
The psychoanalytic metapsychology of schizophrenia

11. Neuropsychoanalysis and schizophrenia   67

12. Early psychoanalytic approaches to understanding schizophrenia   72

13. A review of object relations and severe psychopathology   78

14. Schizophrenic etiology and organismal panic   83

15. The infantile psychotic self   90

16. Flawed ingredients   93

17. Fates of infantile psychotic selves   102

Part III
Psychoanalytic approaches to treating schizophrenia

18. Psychodynamic approaches to treating schizophrenia   109

19. Psychoanalytic treatment of adults suffering from schizophrenia   113

20. Fusing–disconnecting and internalization–externalization cycles   121

21. Development of a steady identification with the "good" analyst   129

22. "Sophisticated" identifications and externalizations   133

23. Permanent elimination of the infantile psychotic self?   137

24. Oedipal issues and superego identifications   140

Part IV
Cultural elements in schizophrenia

25. Schizophrenia and culture   145

26. Causal beliefs related to schizophrenia   148

27. Object relations and culture   152

28. Culture-bound schizophrenia   157

29. Psychoanalysis and syndromes of culture-bound schizophrenia   168

Last words   171

References   175

Index   217

About the authors

Kevin Volkan EdD, PhD, MPH is a founding faculty member and professor of psychology at California State University Channel Islands, where he researches and teaches courses on psychopathology and atypical behaviors, personality theory, as well as Nazi Germany and Eastern philosophy. Dr. Volkan also currently serves on the Graduate Medical Education faculty for the Community Memorial Hospital System in Ventura, CA, where he teaches and conducts research with medical residents, and as an adjunct faculty member for California Lutheran University's clinical psychology doctorate program.

He holds doctorates in clinical and quantitative psychology, is a graduate of the Harvard School of Public Health, and a former Harvard Medical School faculty member and administrator. Dr. Volkan is considered to be an expert on extreme psychopathologies and has testified before the United States Senate on pathological and dangerous fetishes. He has made numerous appearances on television, radio, and podcasts as a psychological expert.

Dr. Volkan's clinical training and experience is in psychoanalytic psychotherapy, though he also has experience using a wide variety of other modalities in clinical practice. He has practiced clinical psychology as a staff psychologist in a state hospital and in private practice.

Dr. Volkan's clients included a diverse population of people representing a wide variety of socioeconomic strata and psychological distress. He has worked with people suffering from drug addiction, neuroses, and personality disorders as well individuals suffering from autism, organic brain injury, and schizophrenia. Dr. Volkan was awarded the *Sustained Superior Accomplishment Award* from the State of California for his clinical work. His current practice is centered upon psychodynamic embodied dreamwork.

Dr. Volkan is the author of *Dancing Among the Maenads: The Psychology of Compulsive Drug Use*, which is one of the few psychoanalytic works examining drug addiction. He has also published a number of papers on psychopathology as well as on psychoanalysis and culture. His current publications include works on delusional misidentification syndromes, hoarding, narcissism, and demonic possession.

Vamık Volkan, MD, DLFAPA is an emeritus professor of psychiatry at the University of Virginia, an emeritus training and supervising analyst at the Washington-Baltimore Psychoanalytic Institute and an emeritus senior Erik Erikson Scholar at the Erikson Institute of the Austen Riggs Center, Stockbridge, Massachusetts. He is the founder and past president of the International Dialogue Initiative and a former president of the Turkish-American Neuropsychiatric Society, the International Society of Political Psychology, the Virginia Psychoanalytic Society, and the American College of Psychoanalysts.

For eighteen of his thirty-nine years at the University of Virginia, Dr. Volkan was the medical director of the university's Blue Ridge Hospital. In 1987, he established the Center for the Study of Mind and Human Interaction (CSMHI). CSMHI applied a growing theoretical and field-proven base of knowledge to issues such as ethnic tension, racism, large-group identity, terrorism, societal trauma, immigration, mourning, transgenerational transmissions, leader-follower relationships, and other aspects of national and international conflict.

Dr. Volkan was an inaugural Yitzhak Rabin Fellow at the Rabin Center, Tel Aviv, Israel; a visiting professor of law, Harvard University, Boston, Massachusetts; a visiting professor of political science at the University of Vienna, Vienna, Austria and at Bahçeşehir University, Istanbul, Turkey. He worked as a visiting professor of psychiatry at three universities in Turkey. In 2006, he was Fulbright/Sigmund Freud-Privatstiftung Visiting Scholar of Psychoanalysis in Vienna, Austria. In 2015, he became a visiting professor at El Bosque University, Bogota, Colombia.

Dr. Volkan holds honorary doctorate degrees from Kuopio University (now called the University of Eastern Finland), Finland; from Ankara University, Turkey; and the Eastern European Psychoanalytic Institute, Russia. He was a member of the Working Group on Terror and Terrorism, International Psychoanalytic Association. He was a temporary consultant to the World Health Organization (WHO) in Albania and Macedonia.

He has received the Nevitt Sanford Award, Elise M. Hayman Award, L. L. Bryce Boyer Award, Margaret Mahler Literature Prize, Hans H. Strupp Award, and American College of Psychoanalysts' Distinguished Officer Award for 2014. He also received the Sigmund Freud Award given by the city of Vienna, Austria in collaboration with the World Council of Psychotherapy and the Mary S. Sigourney Award for 2015. The Sigourney Award was given to him for his role as a "seminal contributor to the application of psychoanalytic thinking to conflicts between countries and cultures," and because "his clinical thinking about the use of object relations theory in primitive mental states has advanced our under-standing of severe personality disorders."

About this book

This book on schizophrenia is born out of the first-hand knowledge of the authors, one of whom has a broad range of experience of working with people suffering from schizophrenia in institutional settings and across cultures using psychodynamic as well as behavioral and psychopharmacological modalities and the other in treating individuals with schizophrenia as a psychoanalyst.

Regardless of the variety of their experience, both authors ground their understanding of schizophrenia from a psychoanalytic view. Unlike other psychological understandings of schizophrenia, the psychoanalytic view is grounded in metapsychology. This is where the subjective view of the analyst or psychotherapist meets the objective scientific understanding of the researcher. Views of the emergent properties of the mind are intertwined with knowledge of neurobiology, evolution, and the structure of the brain. Unlike some Freudians, like George Klein (1976), who saw metapsychology and clinical theory as incompatible, or others who view it as something that is divorced from empirical reality and biology, we take the view postulated by Patricia Kitcher when she says, "… my thesis is that Freud's enduring commitment to metapsychology does not reflect any attachment to particular doctrines, but rather a vision of how various sciences can combine their results to tell us everything we want to know about human mental life" (Kitcher & Wilkes, 1988, p. 102).

This book is our attempt to accomplish this combination in a study of schizophrenia. We acknowledge that the task is difficult. Mainstream research reveals that the causes, prevalence, and treatment of schizophrenia have greatly diverged from psychoanalytic thinking over the last seventy years to the point where there is little common ground. However, the emergence of the field of neuropsychoanalysis gives some hope that psychoanalytic metapsychology and clinical theory may once again provide valuable insight to the mainstream understanding of schizophrenia. We also take hope from the fact that there has always been a small number of clinicians and researchers who have sought to apply psychoanalytic theory and practice to help those suffering from schizophrenia. The sad irony is that this group has been declining just as psychoanalysis has evolved to better understand schizophrenia and provide new possibilities for treating this disorder. Using psychotherapy to treat schizophrenia has become somewhat of a "lost art," at least in the United States. As we shall discuss, the use of psychoanalysis or psychoanalytic psychotherapy is not appropriate for all individuals suffering from schizophrenia.

Part of the problem is that psychoanalytic treatment may not be appropriate for many suffering from schizophrenia, and even for those who may benefit, it may be out of reach due to financial or logistic issues. The challenge for the future, then, is how to meld mainstream understandings of schizophrenia with psychoanalytic insights in order to both inform and improve non-psychoanalytic treatments and/or to produce effective psychoanalytic-based treatments that are more widely applicable to those who suffer the debilitating effects of schizophrenia. Another potential impediment to treating schizophrenia is a lack of recognition about its cultural variants. Psychoanalytic theory can indicate much about what aspects of schizophrenia are common across cultures and where they present unique characteristics. More importantly, psychoanalysis can give an indication of how cultural variations of schizophrenia come about. For future improvement in understanding and treating schizophrenia it will be vitally important to understand the cultural underpinnings and expressions of schizophrenic illness.

While this book will not definitively answer the questions posed by the melding together of mainstream, psychoanalytic, and cultural viewpoints related to schizophrenia, it may provide some guide toward future solutions. For clinicians who currently treat people suffering from schizophrenia, it is our hope that this book will deepen insight into the disorder as well as promote the greater use of psychotherapy and integrated treatments, while increasing sensitivity to cultural variations in schizophrenic disease. Accordingly, this book is divided into four parts.

The first part gives a brief overview and outline of the mainstream understanding of schizophrenia. This includes its epidemiology, possible contributing causes, and treatments. This part also includes discussion of some theories and treatments such as specific focal sepsis that have come and gone, as well as thoughts of alternative treatments and ideas around prevention. With regard to treatment this section also mentions predominating treatment modalities such as psycho-pharmacology, brief and supportive non-analytic psychotherapy, and emerging surgical and neuromodulation treatments.

The second part drills down to focus on general psychoanalytic ideas about schizophrenia, culminating with a focus on problems with early object relations. As shall be noted in this part, this psychoanalytic approach to schizophrenia is not in conflict with mainstream conceptualizations of schizophrenia. Unlike past psychoanalytic conceptions of schizophrenia, we fully acknowledge that the object relations pathology found in individuals suffering from schizophrenia described here may be induced and/or influenced by biological, structural, and environmental causes, as well as by psychological factors.

In *the third part* we look at psychoanalytic treatment and speculate that some schizophrenia, especially unmedicated cases where there are strong psychogenic influences, can be successfully treated by psychoanalysis or psychoanalytic psychotherapy. For cases not amenable to this type of intensive psychotherapy, we speculate that a psychoanalytic understanding of schizophrenia and possibly some types of psychoanalytic therapy could be helpful as a form of adjunct treatment.

In *the fourth part* we take a broad look at schizophrenia and how views of the disorder and the disorder itself are affected by culture. We shall review research on how symptoms of schizophrenia can vary across cultures and how schizophrenia is related to immigration. We will examine how cultural variations can lead to different types of object relations.

It is our hope that the combination of the ideas presented in the four parts of this book will generate insight and understanding of schizophrenic disorders that represent "out of the box" thinking. Hopefully, this will yield new approaches to treating and possibly preventing schizophrenia.

Before beginning, a few notes on terminology and organization are in order. This book is the result of a collaboration between individuals who view schizophrenia from different but overlapping professional viewpoints. This is seen by us as a strength, but we realize that it may cause some confusion in regard to terminology. Although the authors are related (son and father) and have career similarities (both are professors), we carry the viewpoints of the fields we have trained in—psychology and psychiatry, as well as psychoanalytic therapy versus psychoanalysis respectively. These fields overlap to some degree but also have unique viewpoints.

Kevin Volkan is a psychologist, trained in psychoanalytic psychotherapy, but who has practiced using many modalities besides psychoanalysis. He has worked with severe psychopathology but also with people seeking a better understanding of themselves. He has expertise and experience in academic psychology and medicine, using clinical case studies as well as formal statistical hypothesis testing to conduct research in these areas. On the other hand, Vamık Volkan is a psychiatrist and psychoanalyst who has spent his career interacting with patients within the strict milieu of traditional psychoanalytic practice. He has conducted much of his research work using case studies. In writing this book, we have tried to combine and triangulate these different approaches in order to present a richer understanding of schizophrenia.

Nevertheless, some questions related to our different approaches may confuse the reader. For instance, when we refer to psychoanalysis does this include not only traditional psychoanalytic treatment but also psychoanalytic psychotherapy, or even psychotherapy informed by psychoanalysis? The problem is that there is not uniform agreement on the relationship between traditional psychoanalytic treatment and psychoanalytic psychotherapy. For some, psychoanalytic psychotherapy is just psychoanalysis that occurs for fewer sessions in a given week. For others, psychoanalytic psychotherapy forgoes traditional aspects such as the use of the couch and may possibly be more supportive in nature. Add to this that there are varying opinions about how psychoanalysis proper should be conducted, with there being many differences across schools and training centers.

For this work our thought is to minimize the differences between psychiatry and psychology, between psychoanalysis proper and psychoanalytic psychotherapy. We agree on the importance of transference in therapy and both see object relations dynamics at the core of schizophrenic illness. While psychoanalytic psychotherapy may not be as intensive as psychoanalysis proper, it may hold more promise for treating greater numbers of people suffering from schizophrenia, who may not have the financial or emotional resources to engage in traditional psychoanalysis. Although many of the treatment insights put forward here are derived from intensive traditional psychoanalysis, it is hoped that many of these insights can be adapted to psychoanalytic psychotherapy. Likewise, psychoanalytic psychotherapists need to make sure they do not modify psychoanalytic technique to the point where it is no longer effective.

It is realistic to expect that any sort of psychoanalytic therapy will need to be adapted to work with patients suffering schizophrenia who are medicated, or who may undergo some other type of treatment such as neuromodulation or even psychosurgery. It is too early to say what these adaptations will look like or how they will be implemented. It is hoped that this book will provide some impetus for developing such integrated treatments.

Part I

Schizophrenia
Epidemiology, causes, neurobiology, pathophysiology

CHAPTER 1

Introduction and overview
of schizophrenia

Schizophrenia is a term for a mental disorder in which thought and perception are severely impaired. People suffering from schizophrenia have delusional beliefs and, in many instances, these are accompanied by auditory or visual hallucinations. People with schizophrenia display disorganized thinking that can manifest as bizarre personality and behavioral changes that cause impairment in social functioning. The person suffering from schizophrenia demonstrates a marked loss of contact with reality.

The fifth edition of the *Diagnostic and Statistical Manual of Mental Disorders* (DSM V) now understands all psychoses as variants of schizophrenia (American Psychiatric Association, 2013). This schizophrenia spectrum includes schizophrenia, other psychotic disorders, as well as schizotypal disorder (which is generally diagnosed as a personality disorder). The DSM V lists the following schizophrenia spectrum disorders: "schizophrenia, schizophreniform disorder, schizoaffective disorder, delusional disorder, brief psychotic disorder, substance/medication induced psychotic disorder, psychotic disorder due to another medical condition, unspecified schizophrenia and other psychotic disorder" (pp. 87–160).

When we examine these schizophrenia spectrum disorders, it becomes obvious that there are many similarities among the disorders and that they differ only in duration or emphasis on a particular symptom. For instance, schizophrenia, schizophreniform disorder, and brief psychotic disorder differ in terms of duration, while schizophrenia, delusional disorder, and schizoaffective disorder differ in symptomatic content. Some researchers question whether or not schizoaffective disorder is really a separate disorder and not either a variation of schizophrenia or mood disorder (Cheniaux et al., 2008; Marneros, 2007). In fact, scientists and clinicians continue to debate just what constitutes a psychosis (Castle & Morgan, 2008).

Psychotic disorder due to a general medical condition and substance-induced psychotic disorder are both related to psychoses that result from chemical or structural changes in the body. What is clear from all these descriptions is that schizophrenia encompasses all the psychotic characteristics of these disease entities. Another way of saying this is that all these disorders are easily understood as variations of schizophrenia. For that reason, our discussion will focus on schizophrenia.

Positive and negative symptoms of schizophrenia

Schizophrenia presents with symptoms that can be positive, negative, or mixed. The term positive is used to denote symptoms of schizophrenia that have active affective, behavioral, or cognitive components. These symptoms include overt delusions, auditory, visual, and tactile hallucinations, thought disorder, and behavior that is bizarre when compared to normal behavior in the culture where it occurs. Conversely, the term negative denotes schizophrenic symptoms where affective, behavioral, or cognitive functions are muted. These symptoms include a flat affect, alogia, avolition, anhedonia, and impairment of attention. Cognition may also be impaired in those who have the disease with consequences for social functioning (Rossello et al., 2013). Mixed schizophrenic symptoms that include both positive and negative symptoms may also occur (Dion & Dellario, 1988).

Epidemiology of schizophrenia

Schizophrenia typically has an onset in adolescence or young adulthood and most estimates are that approximately 1% of the population is affected (Castle & Morgan, 2008). A review of prevalence data from a large number of geographically diverse studies indicates lifetime prevalence ranging from around 0.2% to almost 1.5% (Simeone et al., 2015). Men are significantly more likely than women to have the disorder (Grignon & Trottier, 2005). While it has commonly been held that prevalence rates for schizophrenia are fairly stable around the world (Nixon & Doody, 2005), some studies are now questioning this dogma, demonstrating that sex, age, ethnicity, and geography are related to its incidence (McGrath, 2006; McGrath et al., 2011). Other studies have shown increasing general rates of schizophrenia (Boydell et al., 2003; Bray et al., 2006) while others have not (Nixon & Doody, 2005; Suvisaari et al., 1999).

There is some debate about whether schizophrenia represents a single disease or many different syndromes. This idea is supported by some studies, like the one by David Garver and his associates (2000) that found that different biological markers are associated with how well patients respond to antipsychotic drugs. The presence of these different biological markers gives support to the idea that schizophrenia may in fact be multiple syndromes rather than a single disease entity. Colin Ross (2006, 2014) argues against the prevailing view that schizophrenia is primarily an inherited biological disorder to be treated solely with medication. He goes on to make the case for viewing the positive symptoms of schizophrenia as being more representative of dissociative identity disorder and proposes a dissociative subtype of schizophrenia. After reviewing many cross-cultural studies of psychoses, Jerome Kroll (2007) concludes that there are so many shared risk factors for psychosis and affective disorders that he questions whether or not there should be a categorical distinction between disorders. In this book, we will present the idea that for some people suffering from schizophrenia, their disease may have primarily psychogenic origins. It may be that this subset of the population of people suffering from schizophrenia might be successfully treated through the intensive application of psychoanalytic based psychotherapy.

Co-morbidity and mortality

People who suffer from schizophrenia often suffer from other mental health issues such as anxiety disorders, depression, and substance abuse, as well as from physical problems related to cardiovascular, oral, respiratory, and endocrine pathology (Laursen, 2019; Laursen et al., 2012). A number of researchers have pointed out that people who suffer from schizophrenia may be at higher risk from health problems that stem from unhealthy behavior patterns related to smoking, eating, and sexual behaviors, which are preventable (Arnaiz et al., 2011; Chwastiak & Tek, 2009; Findlay, 2012; Trudeau et al., 2018).

As might be expected, the presence of comorbid conditions is associated with worse symptoms, treatment outcomes, and social functioning (Pratt, 2012; Sim, Chan et al., 2006; Sim, Chua et al., 2006). People who suffer from schizophrenia often have social dysfunction. They are more likely to be unemployed, poor, and homeless. Unfortunately, this leads to decreased life expectancy with some estimates as much as ten to twelve years less than people who do not suffer from schizophrenia (S. Brown et al., 2000). Other studies have shown that on average individuals with schizophrenia live about thirty-six years after diagnosis and that this number is decreasing (Capasso et al., 2008; Saha et al., 2007).

After reviewing more than forty thousand studies Stefan Leucht and colleagues (2007) concluded that individuals suffering from schizophrenia in developed nations have increased rates of HIV, hepatitis, osteoporosis, sensitivity to pain, sexual dysfunction, obstetric complications, cardiovascular diseases, obesity, diabetes, dental problems, and polydipsia when compared to the general population. Interestingly, people suffering from schizophrenia were found to have lower rates of rheumatoid arthritis and cancer. The authors conclude that many of these medical problems may be related to the treatment delivered by health services as well as the social stigma attached to the disease.

Long-term use of antipsychotic medication is also suspected of decreasing life expectancy in people suffering from schizophrenia (Fors et al., 2007; Healy, 2006; Joukamaa et al., 2006). Antipsychotic medications may increase mortality among individuals suffering from schizophrenia by contributing to obesity, hyperglycemia, diabetes mellitus, and dyslipidemia (Casey et al., 2004; Robinson, 2008). One study reported that people suffering from schizophrenia who use antipsychotic medication were five times more likely to suffer from a heart attack than healthy controls (Enger et al., 2004). Suicide is found more often in people suffering from schizophrenia with males having higher rates of mortality (Lester, 2007). This finding is seen across cultures and may explain the higher prevalence of schizophrenia among females in some areas (Ran et al., 2007).

CHAPTER 2

Causes of schizophrenia

It is still not known what causes schizophrenia and how it develops. Also, it is not yet clear that schizophrenia is a unitary disorder or a number of related syndromes. Nevertheless, researchers are cautiously optimistic that we will soon have some answers regarding the etiology of this disease (Schwab & Wildenauer, 2008). While generally thought to be a disease of the brain, studies suggest that genetics, early environment, psychological, and social processes are important contributory factors to its development (K. Dean et al., 2003; Gilmore, 2010). Indeed, there is recent support for the older idea of psychogenic causes or contributions to the development of the disease. As Henrik Lublin and Jonas Eberhard (2008) put it:

> Basic research into the mechanisms behind the disorder suggest that the possibility of psychogenesis still appears to have some validity, although we may never entirely come to understand the relationships and possible interactions between the environmental and genetic risks ... We know that, like many other disorders, there are susceptible individuals who appear to have inherited a number of genetic traits, each of which is also present in the general population, but which, together, render that individual vulnerable to schizophrenia. These include neurodevelopmental genes—but

they are by no means the whole story ... there is still much work to do on our understanding of the contribution of early environmental "insults" such as prenatal infections, maternal malnutrition, substance abuse, and obstetric complications ... (p. v)

E. Fuller Torrey and colleagues (2012) report on a number of causative risk factors for schizophrenia. Having a mother with schizophrenia raises risk of the disorder 9.3 times, while having a father or sibling with the disorder raises risk 7.2 times. However, other risk factors abound. Being the offspring of an immigrant increases risk of schizophrenia 4.5 times while being an immigrant from certain countries increases the risk 2.7 times. T. gondii infection also results in a 2.7 times greater risk. Being born or raised in an urban setting increases risk 2.2–2.8 times, while cannabis use, minor physical abnormalities, and having a father over fifty-five at time of birth results in around 2 times the risk. The authors found other risk factors to have minor impacts, increasing the risk of schizophrenia 1–1.7 times. These factors include traumatic brain injury, being sexually abused as a child, complications during birth, having a father forty-five or older at birth, season of birth, having specific genetic variations, and maternal exposure to the flu. We will discuss some of these factors below and also attempt to explain that at least one form of schizophrenia has primarily psychogenic origins related to early object relations pathology, and that this type of schizophrenia may respond well to intensive psychotherapy.

Genetics of schizophrenia

There is a tremendous amount of research on the genetics of schizophrenia, and a great deal of progress has been made in understanding the genetics underlying the disorder (Mulle, 2012). Here we will present some highlights from recent genetic research that is likely to have relevance to future understanding and treatment of schizophrenia.

It is well known that schizophrenia has been shown to have a strong genetic component. Having first-degree relatives with the disorder greatly increases the risk of developing schizophrenia and schizophrenia spectrum disorders. Heritability of schizophrenia and schizophrenia spectrum disorders, as demonstrated by twin studies, is quite high, ranging from 70–80% (Hilker et al., 2018). However, as indicated in a review by Patrick Sullivan and his colleagues (2012), the heritability of schizophrenia is complicated and does not follow simple Mendelian inheritance patterns. This review shows that there are some very rare inherited genetic structural variations that are thought to increase risk, but these do not directly cause schizophrenia. Instead, heritability of schizophrenia and schizophrenia spectrum disorders are polygenically spread across a number of loci. Genes associated with calcium channels that regulate neuronal excitability, as well as neurogranin, which may act as a calcium sensor, have been associated with schizophrenia, suggesting that calcium biology in the brain may be a fruitful area of schizophrenia research. The strongest association to schizophrenia was found in the major histocompatibility complex (MHC) gene region. This region is related to immunity, autoimmunity, and synaptic pruning. The involvement of this genetic region supports research demonstrating a relationship between autoimmunity, inter-uterine infection, synaptic pruning (Keshavan et al., 2020), viral infection, and schizophrenia. A gene associated with miR-137, which is a short non-coding RNA molecule that is involved in the regulation of neuronal development and is highly expressed in the synapses in the cortex and hippocampus, was also found to be associated with schizophrenia.

Copy number variation (CNV) in the human genome has been found to be associated with schizophrenia (Gulsuner & McClellan, 2015). This occurs when the number of copies or repeats of a specific gene or part of the genome varies from person to person. CNVs can consist of duplications or deletions and can manifest as short or long repeats and can be classified as de novo (newly acquired) or inherited (K. W. Lee et al., 2012). It is thought 4.8–9.5% of the human genome consists of CNVs and that these contribute to natural human genetic variation (McCarroll & Altshuler, 2007; Zarrei et al., 2015). It is not fully understood how CNVs affect human health. Besides schizophrenia, CNVs may possibly be associated with a number of other diseases and syndromes including Alzheimer's disease, Angelman syndrome, anxiety disorder, attention-deficit/hyperactivity disorder, autism spectrum disorders, some cancers, DiGeorge syndrome, glomerulonephritis, hypercholesterolemia, lipodystrophy, Parkinson disease, Prader-Willi syndrome, psoriasis, Smith–Magenis syndrome, William's syndrome, as well as non-responsiveness to antidepressant medication and an increase in codeine toxicity (Ellenbroek & Youn, 2016; Heckel et al., 2015; Heng, 2017; Huang, 2019; Lanktree et al., 2010; McCarroll & Altshuler, 2007; Shao et al., 2019; Zhang et al., 2009).

In a small number of people suffering from schizophrenia few CNVs with large phenotypic effects are the primary contributing factor to the disorder; in other schizophrenia sufferers there may be many CNVs that have more minor effects on phenotype (Caseras et al., 2021; Clair, 2013; Gulsuner & McClellan, 2015; Thygesen et al., 2020). CNVs are not fully penetrant in schizophrenia meaning that not all people with CNVs develop the disorder (Stefansson et al., 2014). CNVs in people suffering from schizophrenia have been found to be associated with cognition, cortical thickness, corticogenesis, cytokine receptors, major histocompatibility complex, neurogenesis, neuronal development and regeneration, oligodendrocyte progenitor expression and differentiation, among many other functions. These CNVs demonstrate that genes involved in the development of the brain and its structures as well as autoimmunity and inflammation have a role in the development of schizophrenic illness. The wide variation of CNVs suggests that there may be a number of different pathways leading to the genesis of schizophrenic disorder (K. W. Lee et al., 2012; Thygesen et al., 2020).

Recent research by Yang Zhenxing and associates (2018) indicates that mutations at genetic loci related to schizophrenia are heterogenous, with a relatively weak contribution of any single mutation. Other studies have sought to understand how the large number of genes involved with schizophrenia contributes to the development of the disease. A study by Antonio Pardiñas and his associates (2018) using genetic data from over 11,000 cases of schizophrenia and over 24,000 control subjects, combined with a meta-analysis of data from previous studies, revealed 50 novel loci related to schizophrenia and 145 loci overall. The authors were able to identify 33 candidate genes within 33 loci that are speculated to have some direct causal relationship to schizophrenia. This study importantly indicates that loss of function (LoF) intolerant genes (i.e. gene variants that cause a loss of function among genes that have a critical function) account for 30% of the SNP (single nucleotide polymorphisms)-based heritability of schizophrenia. Additionally, six gene sets representing molecular, physiological, and behavioral pathways related to the pathogenesis of schizophrenia were uncovered. The study also found that the persistence of gene variants related to schizophrenia is not likely subject to high selection pressure, but to background selection (BGS). This explains how schizophrenia can persist in human populations even though people suffering from schizophrenia are less likely to have children than those who do not suffer from the disorder.

An important consideration when examining the genetic contribution to schizophrenia is gender. A recent genome-wide association study analyzing data from close to 200,000 patients and summarizing the contributions from over 100 authors (Blokland et al., 2021), found differences between males and females in the genetic underpinnings of schizophrenia. Nearly a dozen single nucleotide polymorphisms (SNPs) were found that differed between men and women diagnosed with one of three severe mental illnesses; bipolar disorder, depressive affect, and schizophrenia. SNPs associated with an increase in one disorder were found in some cases to be associated with a decrease in the same disorder, or others with disorders in the opposite gender. The SNPs involved were related to immune, neuronal, and vascular developmental pathways. This study indicates that it is essential for sex-based differences to be considered in genetic studies and treatments arising from genetic research.

This is just a quick survey of the genetic research on schizophrenia. This is a very active area of inquiry that is likely to continue to illuminate the neurobiology and neurostructural correlates of schizophrenia, leading to improved understanding and treatments.

Epigenetics of schizophrenia

Genetics has been shown to be related to early brain development; however, how and when genes are expressed may be related to the circumstances in which the development of the brain takes place. As will be discussed, a number of postnatal risk factors such as infection, exposure to drugs, etc., can increase the risk of schizophrenia. Also, prenatal factors such as maternal infection, obstetric complications, and maternal nutrition can increase the likelihood of schizophrenia occurring in offspring (Eyles, 2021). While genetics operates primarily through modification of DNA nucleotide sequences via natural selection and mutation, epigenetics examines how genes are expressed without any changes in the underlying DNA sequences. The field of epigenetics attempts to examine how a person's experiences (via their behavior and their environment), as well as the experiences of previous generations, can affect genetic expression in individuals. The regulation of genetic expression is typically accomplished through DNA methylation, chromatin (histone) modification, and non-coding micro RNAs (Gürel et al., 2020). DNA methylation is where methyl (CH_3) groups are added to the C5 position of cytosine in the DNA molecule to form 5-methylcytosine. Gene expression is then regulated through proteins involved in gene repression or by the inhibition of DNA transcription factors (Gong & Xu, 2017; Jobe & Zhao, 2017; Mateen et al., 2017). Chromatin consists of DNA and core histone proteins that act to package DNA to fit into the nucleus. This is accomplished by spooling the DNA around the histone proteins that are subject to post-translational modification by acetylation, phosphorylation, and methylation. These modifications affect the rate of gene transcription by regulating physical access to the gene. This can be thought of as how tightly the DNA is wrapped around the histone (Rumbaugh & Miller, 2011). Non-coding micro RNAs (miRNAs) are short oligonucleotides consisting of around 22 bases. These miRNAs work by inhibiting translation of messenger RNA (mRNA), which leaves the nucleus and is read (translated) by ribosomes to make proteins. This inhibition of translation by miRNAs is accomplished through degradation of mRNA or through suppression of its translation. These properties allow miRNAs to regulate the expression of multiple proteins simultaneously and therefore make them excellent regulators of complex networks of genes (Noack & Calegari, 2014). These epigenetic changes to gene expression can occur under the influence of physiological, behavioral, and environmental stimuli (Moore et al., 2013).

Given that epigenetics has been shown to play a role in cognition, interneuron migration and maturation, memory, neuronal activity, neurogenesis, as well as neurodegeneration and neuroprotection (Adam & Harwell, 2020; Bayraktar & Kreutz, 2018; J.-Y. Hwang et al., 2017; Zimmer-Bensch, 2018), it is not surprising that epigenetics is associated with schizophrenia.

Lukasz Smigielski and his colleagues (2020) have recently conducted a systematic review of epigenetic mechanisms involved with schizophrenia. The authors examined 152 studies which studied the association of DNA methylation, histone modification, and miRNAs to schizophrenic illness. The studies under review totaled 14,139 cases diagnosed with schizophrenia or schizophrenia spectrum disorders and 13,574 normal control subjects. All three epigenetic mechanisms were found to be associated with schizophrenia. Global methylation was found to be ambiguously related to schizophrenia with some studies reporting hyper methylation, while other studies reported lower levels of, or no differences in, methylation. When specific genes related to the regulation of dopamine, serotonin, gamma-aminobutyric acid, and neurotrophin were studied there were varying levels of evidence supporting altered DNA methylation. Genome-wide methylation studies showed differences in methylation sites between those with schizophrenic disorders and control subjects. Functional annotation, which identifies tissue-specific variation in methylation, turned up differences in neuroinflammation and immune functions, supporting a link between schizophrenia and dysregulated immunity. There were similar functional annotation findings for methylation differences in genes related to mitochondrial deficits, aberrant neurotransmitter signaling, neurogenesis, and neurodevelopment. Two studies demonstrated an increase in histone H3K9 di-methylation, which prevents activation of gene expression. In people suffering from schizophrenia and schizophrenia spectrum disorders the hypothesis that miRNA is dysregulated was generally supported. There are a number of miRNAs which may be biomarkers for schizophrenia but the exact roles for many are still unclear. The review found a number of other variables to be associated with epigenetic mechanisms including age, alcohol use, anti-psychotic medication, body mass index, brain anatomy or function, cognition, family history of schizophrenic illness, disease onset, gender, genotype, illness duration, tobacco use, and symptomology. The authors suggest "… that numerous disease-related, unspecific, and environmental conditions influence the epigenetic landscape" (p. 1741). They go on to propose that in the future longitudinal studies be conducted that look at epigenetic changes before and after the onset of psychosis. With regards to treatment, drugs that modulate epigenetic signaling have potential as thera-peutics. It is suggested that histone demethylase inhibitors (HMT), histone deacetylase inhibitors (HDAC), and DNA methyltransferase inhibitors (DNMT) have potential as a new class of medication for treating schizophrenia. The authors conclude their review by stating, "Despite the variability of results examined, this systematic review provides support for the view that epigenetic mechanisms differentiate healthy controls from cases with schizophrenia and related psychotic disorders" (p. 1742).

Another review by Çevik Gürel and associates (2020) came to similar conclusions. This study similarly reviewed research that demonstrated that various antipsychotic medications as well as valproic acid induce epigenetic changes. The authors report that there are a few methylation related biomarkers that are significantly higher in the blood of patients suffering from schizophrenia compared to controls. These biomarkers may have potential as diagnostic tools.

Richetto and Meyer (2020) in another study conclude that a substantial quantity of the epigenetic changes related to schizo-phrenia are acquired through environmental factors that manifest as "molecular scars" (p. 219). These molecular scars can influence brain functioning and some can be transmitted across generations while others can affect brain functions throughout the life span. These environmental factors can be present in the pre-, peri-, and postnatal periods and have been shown to have a negative impact on early brain development and subsequent development of schizophrenia. The environmental factors include maternal alcohol consumption, chemical exposure, drug use, immune activation/infection during pregnancy, malnourishment, psychiatric disorders, and stress. Maternal stress and immune activation are perhaps the most common environ-mental factors related to the development of schizophrenia in offspring (Cattane et al., 2020).

In theory, abnormal epigenetic gene expression is reversible; therefore, targeting the effects of environmental factors may lead to normative changes in gene expression. This supports the idea that use of non-pharmacological treatments such as psychotherapy, which targets the effects of environmental insults, could be useful in treating people suffering from schizophrenia.

Childhood abuse, trauma, and schizophrenia

The association between childhood abuse and subsequent diagnosis of schizophrenia is complicated. There are a number of studies that indicate a relationship between childhood abuse and schizophrenia. One study by John Read and his coworkers (2003) found that abuse as a child (sexual and physical) was significantly related to hallucinations, but not delusions, thought disorders, or negative symptoms among community mental health center clients. Child abuse and subsequent abuse as an adult predicted hallucinations, delusions, and thought disorders.

John Read and colleagues (2005) also completed a systematic review of the literature. They found a strong causal association between child physical and sexual abuse, and schizophrenic symptoms, especially hallucinations. This review also supports the idea of a dosage effect with higher levels of abuse being associated with more severe psychotic symptoms. The authors conclude that many severe mental illnesses, including schizophrenia as well as post-traumatic stress syndrome and other diagnoses related to dissociation (e.g. borderline personality disorder and dissociative disorders) can be understood as adaptive responses to early childhood trauma that are subsequently maladaptive in adults. This fits with the idea that child abuse contributes to a spectrum of dissociation with phenomena such as splitting defenses at the milder end and dissociative identity disorder and schizophrenia (severe dissociation) at the other end. In this rubric, the voices hallucinated by people suffering from schizophrenia can been understood as a dissociated aspect of personality akin to an "alter" in dissociative identity disorder. Throughout history people suffering from schizophrenia have been thought to be "possessed by demons" that can be understood as disassociated objects. It no surprise that people thought to be "possessed," like those suffering from schizophrenia, are highly likely to have been abused as children (K. Volkan, 2020b).

Ilse Janssen, along with his colleagues (2004), in a study of over 4000 subjects drawn from a general population, found that people who had suffered abuse as a child were 7.3 times more likely to develop positive schizophrenic symptoms compared to those who had not been subjected to abuse as a child, after adjustment for confounding. This study also demonstrated a dose-effect with those having experienced higher levels of abuse having more severe psychotic symptoms. Those subjects with the highest frequency of abuse as children were found to be 30 times more likely to have psychotic symptoms than those who were not abused.

While many studies show a strong association between childhood sexual and physical abuse and schizophrenia, other studies have found conflicting results. Josie Spataro and associates (2004), in a study of 1612 sexually abused children, found significant rates of affective disorders, anxiety disorders, childhood mental disorders, and personality disorders, but not schizophrenia. Paul Mullen (2005) states that the associations in many studies were related to schizophrenic symptoms but not fully diagnosable schizophrenic disorder.

In a series of studies Paul Lysaker and colleagues (2001, 2004, 2005) found that childhood sexual abuse victims who were later diagnosed with schizophrenia spectrum disorders reported higher levels of psychotic symptoms, as well as poorer psychosocial functioning and participation in vocational rehabilitation. The subjects who suffered from schizophrenia were also more likely to perform worse in tests of executive function and have higher levels of hallucinations and anxiety. A similar study found that adult patients diagnosed with schizophrenia (but not having acute psychotic episodes) had increased disability, functional impairment in overall behavior, social role performance, and global functioning (i.e., how well an individual deals with psychological and social problems in living as derived from a combination of the other measures). In a study by Alexei Gil and associates (2009), higher emotional abuse was associated with impaired overall behavioral functioning and higher emotional neglect was associated with a decrease in global functioning. Physical neglect was associated with the subjects' overall ability to function as adults. There was no association found between sexual and physical abuse and schizophrenia.

Other research by Franck Schürhoff and his coworkers (2009) found a strong correlation between childhood trauma and positive schizotypal tendencies among unaffected first-degree relatives of people suffering from schizophrenia. A correlation between childhood trauma and bipolar tendencies was not found among the relatives of subjects with bipolar disorder. In a study conducted by Matthias Vogel and associates (2011) that compared non-psychotic and adult subjects suffering from schizophrenia, the researchers found that childhood abuse was related to non-psychotic disorders while neglect was related to development of schizophrenia. It was thought that childhood abuse can cause different symptoms in adults with psychotic and non-psychotic disorders. In a study of patients suffering from schizophrenia completed by Katie Ashcroft and her colleagues (2012), they found that those with persecutory delusions reported significantly more emotional abuse than those patients without these delusions. There was no difference in these two groups with regard to total trauma, physical abuse, physical neglect, and sexual abuse. Another study by Bethany Leonhardt and her coworkers (2015) found that patients suffering from schizophrenia with increased awareness and concomitant increased distress were more likely to have experienced abuse as children. Other research done by Deanna Kelly and colleagues (2016) found a positive relationship between men and women diagnosed with schizophrenic and schizoaffective disorders and childhood abuse. Women who were sexually abused as children were more likely to show significantly more psychotic and depressive symptoms compared to women without childhood trauma and men with and without childhood trauma. Another study conducted by Hwigon Kim and colleagues (2018) examined the relationship between childhood trauma and delusions and hallucinations among 42 subjects diagnosed with schizophrenia. Delusions of reference, persecutory delusions, and delusions of being controlled were found to be related to childhood emotional abuse. Childhood abuse and neglect were not found to be related to hallucinations.

A recent study completed by Karolina Rokita and colleagues (2020) found that patients suffering from schizophrenia were significantly more likely to recall childhood trauma and scored lower on social-cognitive measures and measures of parental bonding. Physical neglect was the strongest predictor of impairment in the ability to recognize emotions in others. Good bonding with parents attenuated the impact of childhood trauma and impairment in emotional recognition. The fact that child abuse can cause issues that contribute to a person developing schizophrenia supports the notion that in some cases schizophrenia may have psychogenic origins that can be treated with psychotherapy.

Overall, the preponderance of the evidence is that there is a relationship between childhood abuse and schizophrenic symptoms. A dose-effect relationship has been demonstrated in many studies where an increase in child abuse leads to worse schizophrenic symptoms and negative effects of the disorder. Emotional abuse seems to show a relationship to schizophrenic symptoms in many studies, while the specific contributions of neglect and sexual abuse to the development of schizophrenia have been mixed. Likewise, the relationship between child abuse and the development of delusions and hallucinations is mixed, with some studies reporting a positive association with these symptoms and others not. More research with large populations examining different types of specific types of child abuse and trauma with schizophrenia is in order. Given what is known, however, clinicians working with those suffering from schizophrenia would do well to consider the possibility and effects of child abuse among those they are treating.

Drug abuse and schizophrenia

While both schizophrenia and drug abuse typically have onset in adolescence or young adulthood the relationship between them is not clear. It may be that vulnerability to substance abuse disorders and schizophrenia involves a similar neurobiological substrate (Murray et al., 2003; Zullino et al., 2010). Some studies suggest that drug abuse may in fact be causally related to later development of schizophrenia. This is especially likely for dopaminergic substances such as amphetamines, cocaine, and cannabis (Tsapakis et al., 2003; Weiser et al., 2003). Other studies suggest that drug use among people suffering from schizophrenia may be related to emotional abuse and that they use drugs mainly for social reasons (Gearon et al., 2001). Genetically vulnerable individuals who have experienced high stress events and who use drugs may be especially at risk for developing schizophrenia (P. Miller et al., 2001). Nevertheless, there is also evidence that substance abusers with schizophrenia do not suffer from increased neuropsychological impairments and exhibit fewer negative symptoms (Joyal et al., 2003).

Cannabis use has been especially linked to schizophrenia in a number of studies (Roser, 2019). Cannabis is thought to double the risk of developing schizophrenia in vulnerable people. Heavier dosage and early age of use are associated with increased risk (Ortiz-Medina et al., 2018). A large study of young adults aged eighteen to thirty-four which looked at risk factors for schizophrenia found that a diagnosis of schizophrenia was associated with a history of trauma, a family history of drug problems, bisexuality, use of cannabis, cigarettes and alcohol, as well as drug use before the age of sixteen. The majority of people who developed schizophrenia used both cannabis and cigarettes. The researchers concluded that there was little support for an association between cannabis use and the development of schizophrenia after adjusting for history of trauma, sexual orientation, use of other substances, and family history of substance use. Cigarette use in adolescence and other drug use was associated with schizophrenia. This study demonstrates the importance of including potentially confounding factors when researching the association between cannabis use and schizophrenia (Ryan et al., 2020). These results contradict a slightly earlier study that used a genetic approach to demonstrate a causal relationship between cannabis use and schizophrenia even when accounting for cigarette smoking (Vaucher et al., 2018). As more locations legalize cannabis use the need for research to clarify the causal association between cannabis use and schizophrenia becomes increasingly important. Until more is known it would remain prudent for clinicians to advise against the use of cannabis before or during adolescence and young adulthood, especially if other risk factors are present and there is a family history of schizophrenia. Some good news is that patients suffering a first episode of psychosis, who then stopped using cannabis, were able to reverse the worsening of schizophrenic symptoms that could be attributed to cannabis use. This suggests that intervention efforts aimed at getting patients with first episode psychotic breaks, and perhaps individuals with more established schizophrenia, to stop using cannabis could reduce the severity of the disease (Setién-Suero et al., 2019).

The role of stress, geography, and birth conditions

Stress may play a role in the development of schizophrenic disease (Gomes & Grace, 2018). Immigration and migration, which are highly stressful, are known to increase risk of schizophrenia (Dykxhoorn et al., 2019; Henssler et al., 2020). Elevated prevalence of schizo-phrenia has been demonstrated in both current and past immigrant populations (Fearon et al., 2006; Henssler et al., 2020; Leão et al., 2006; Shekunov, 2016). We will discuss this in more detail in a later chapter. Second generation immigrants are also at increased risk for schizophrenia (Bhugra, 2000). A study of Holocaust survivors demonstrated that prenatal and early life exposure to adversity resulted in a significantly greater risk of developing schizophrenia (Butler et al., 1994).

Researchers have shown a relationship between prevalence of schizophrenia and latitude (Saha, Chant, et al., 2006). Although a difference in rates of schizophrenia has been noted between developed and developing nations (Bresnahan et al., 2003) and a higher incidence of schizophrenia has been associated with developed nations, economic status of a country by itself was not predictive of incidence of the disease (Saha, Welham, et al., 2006). However, inequality among the most socio-economically deprived has been associated with an increased incidence of schizophrenia (Peltzer, 1999).

Some research has suggested that season of birth may be related to the development of schizophrenia later in life. This seasonality may be a proxy for stress as well as infection status, maternal hormone levels, sperm quality, etc. (Tochigi et al., 2004). Other research has shown that a mother's pregnancy and birth conditions themselves have a moderate association with the development of schizophrenia in her offspring. Lack of contact with health care professionals, premature birth, infection with influenza virus, preeclampsia, hemorrhage during birth, manual extraction of the baby during delivery, and maternal sepsis during childbirth and the puerperium, all increased the risk of subsequent development of schizophrenia in the offspring. Interestingly, the greatest risk shown in this study was from infection of the mother by the influenza virus (Byrne et al., 2007). Severe obstetric complications have been shown to be related to lower IQ and the development of schizophrenia. It is thought that obstetric complications should be considered as a neurodevelopmental risk factor for severe mental illness (Wortinger et al., 2020).

Infectious disease as a cause of schizophrenia

A number of infectious agents have been theorized to cause or trigger the onset of schizophrenia. This theory gained some prominence in the twentieth century, with even prominent physicians such as Karl Menninger (1919a, 1919b, 1920, 1922, 1926, 1928) noting the increase in cases of psychosis after the influenza pandemic of 1918 (Hendrick, 1928). Around the turn of the century the so-called "focal sepsis" theory of mental illness became popular in Europe and the United States. Psychiatrists were eager to identify and treat (often through surgery) mental illness through the eradication of infection just as physicians were doing successfully in many other areas of medicine. The use of surgical eradication of bacteria to cure mental illness is documented by Andrew Scull in the book *Madhouse: A Tragic Tale of Megalomania and Modern Medicine* (2005).

In the early twentieth century Henry Cotton, a psychiatrist and director of a mental hospital in New Jersey, promoted the surgical removal of body parts in order to "remove" the infection that he was certain caused psychosis and other mental illness in his patients. The organs Dr. Cotton ordered removed included the cervix, gall bladder, ovaries, sinuses, spleen, stomach, teeth, testicles, and tonsils. Dr. Cotton was especially worried about the colon and this organ was often the target of his infection elimination surgery. Many hundreds of patients underwent unnecessary and dangerous surgeries (in pre-antibiotic times) because of Dr. Cotton's obsession about the infectious causation of severe mental disease. Dr. Cotton reported very high success rates, upwards of 85%. However, these rates were largely anecdotal, and he did not mention the very high rates of morbidity from the surgeries, not to mention their debilitating effects among the survivors (ironically, most morbidity and mortality from the surgeries were due to postoperative infections that were common in the pre-antibiotic era). Dr. Cotton even had his sons' teeth removed in order to prevent them from being infected as a preventative measure to insure their mental health. He also subjected his youngest son to abdominal surgery as a prophylaxis against mental illness and eventually convinced his wife to have all her teeth removed.

Dr. Cotton's positive results for treating mental disease through focal sepsis could not be replicated by other researchers. Two very damning reviews of his research and methods were completed, but never disseminated. While Dr. Cotton's work was investigated and prominent psychiatrists involved with the investigation knew the uselessness of his treatment methods, his career remained largely unaffected. He continued in his post until his retirement, after which there was a marked reduction at least in abdominal surgery. The removal of focal sepsis as a treatment for mental disease did not fall out of favor until other treatments such as lobotomy came on the scene (Scull, 2005).

Because of clinicians like Cotton, infection as a causative factor in schizophrenia and psychoses fell out of favor. However, using much more sensitive tools, medicine is turning again to this line of research. In a quantitative review Stéphane Potvin and her colleagues (2008) proposed that there may indeed be infectious agents that directly affect the development of schizophrenia, or trigger autoimmune reactions that may be related to the disorder. Potential schizophregenic infectious agents include coronaviruses, cytomegalovirus, herpes simplex virus, and Toxoplasma gondii (a parasitic protozoa commonly found in house cats), as well as influenza viruses. A study conducted by Faith Dickerson and her associates (Dickerson et al., 2006) found a relationship between the presence of antibodies to cytomegalovirus and "deficit" schizophrenia (i.e. schizophrenia with a preponderance of negative symptoms). This study did not find any relationships between other viruses and schizophrenia.

Infection with Toxoplasma gondii (T. gondii) has long been suspected of contributing to the development of schizophrenia and has also been associated with increased mortality among schizophrenia sufferers (Dickerson et al., 2007). T. gondii is a neurotropic protozoan parasite that infects over a billion people around the world. Most people do not notice any ill effects from the parasite although it can cause complications in pregnancy including miscarriage, premature labor, stillbirth, and fetal abnormalities (Rashno et al., 2019). There is evidence that T. gondii has an affinity for neural tissue. Two epidemiological studies have found a relationship between increased prevalence of T. gondii antibodies and increased risk of glioma (Hodge et al., 2021). There have been numerous studies showing a relationship between T. gondii infection and risk for schizophrenia (Dickerson et al., 2007; Xiao et al., 2018). Best estimates from numerous studies indicate that T. gondii infection results in an almost 2.7 times increase in risk for developing schizophrenia compared to non-infected people (Torrey et al., 2012). A genome-wide association study found a number of genes associated with T. gondii infection were related to neurodevelopment and psychiatric disorders, especially schizophrenia (A.W. Wang et al., 2019). David Niebuhr and colleagues (2008) found a significant positive association between T. gondii antibodies and diagnosis of schizophrenia among military personnel. Interestingly, T. gondii infection has been shown to be related to a number of risk-taking behaviors ranging from dangerous driving, suicide attempts, and risky sexual pursuits (Flegr & Kuba, 2016; Sutterland et al., 2019). It may be that T. gondii-induced neuronal changes that can cause an escalation in risk-taking behavior may be related to an increased risk of developing schizophrenia.

Studies in Sweden found that viral infection of the central nervous system conferred a slight increased risk of developing schizophrenia and non-affective psychoses while bacterial infection did not. The later development of psychotic illness was specifically associated with the mumps or cytomegalovirus. The authors concluded that there was an association of severe viral central nervous system infection in childhood to viruses that can invade the actual brain tissue (Dalman et al., 2008; Khandaker et al., 2012). Some studies have suggested that the interaction of genes known to have variations related to schizophrenia and viral infection could increase the likelihood of schizophrenia (Beraki et al., 2005).

Human respiratory coronaviruses are also known to infect the nervous system. Recently, there has been speculation that people with schizophrenia may have more risk of contracting COVID-19 (Fonseca et al., 2020; Kozloff et al., 2020). Therefore, it is possible that there could be a future increase in cases of schizophrenia as a result of COVID-19 virus infection. It is also possible that increase in cases of schizophrenia after COVID-19 infection could be related to the social and psychological stress and upheaval caused by the pandemic (Cowan, 2020; Fierini et al., 2020; Watson et al., 2021; Zandifar & Badrfam, 2020).

In a recent study Maxime Taquet and colleagues (2021) reviewed retrospective cohort studies which examined psychiatric diagnoses over

62,000 COVID-19 cases from 14–90 days post-COVID diagnosis. This review demonstrated that recently diagnosed COVID-19 patients had over 1.5 times greater risk for anxiety, insomnia, and dementia compared to controls who had been diagnosed with influenza or other respiratory infections. Approximately 18% of those diagnosed with COVID-19 had psychiatric issues. While this review did not find an increased risk specifically for schizophrenia, it did indicate that the virus could affect the brain a relatively short time after COVID-19 diagnosis.

Cameron Watson and his colleagues (2021) report that there have been many historical associations reported between viral infections and subsequent development of psychosis. They note that hundreds of acute post influenza cases of psychosis were reported during and after the 1918 Spanish influenza pandemic. They mention that Karl Menninger (1919a, 1919b, 1920, 1922, 1926, 1928) wrote extensively about cohorts of patients who presented with schizophrenia-like illness after suffering from influenza. Menninger noted that some patients who suffered from schizophrenia-like illness after suffering from influenza actually made a full recovery, unlike the neurocognitive decline that was typically seen in patients suffering from schizophrenia.

More recently, other studies have reported increased cases of schizophrenia-like illness related to viral severe acute respiratory syndrome (SARS) and Middle East respiratory syndrome (MERS) infection. It was not clear whether this illness was due to a virus or the treatment for the viral condition. Watson and his colleagues go on to list a number of studies that show a correlational association between schizophrenia and COVID-19. Nevertheless, causal inferences about COVID-19 and schizophrenia are difficult to demonstrate. It is unclear whether schizophrenia in COVID-19 patients is induced directly by the virus acting on the brain, systemic inflammation, autoimmunity, vascular pathologies, or other disease and iatrogenic factors. These factors have also been noted by other researchers as well as the fact that these conditions can be negatively affected by social and economic impairments caused by the pandemic (Rogers et al., 2020). It is possible that these psycho-social-economic stressors can result in so-called "stress-incubation," whereby people susceptible to schizophrenia may be at higher risk for having a psychotic break under stressful conditions (Fierini et al., 2020).

Prefrontal cortical structures in the brain have been found to be different among people with schizophrenia depending upon herpes simplex virus 1 (HSV-l) seropositivity (Prasad et al., 2007a). On first diagnosis, patients suffering from schizophrenic and schizoaffective disorders who were exposed to HSV-1 had decreased gray matter in the dorsolateral prefrontal cortex and anterior cingulate cortex when compared to patients suffering from schizophrenia who were not exposed to HSV-1. Differences in brain structure that were related to HSV-1 exposure were not found among healthy control subjects. This suggests that HSV-1 exposure may be related to changes in brain morphology commonly associated with schizophrenia, independent of medication use, comorbid chronic illness, and substance abuse. This can be seen in brain scans produced by Prasad et al. (2007b).

Animal models have demonstrated the theoretical possibility of prenatal induced schizophrenia in offspring through a mimicked viral infection (Moreno et al., 2011). Studies in humans have suggested that prenatal exposure to infectious agents appear to contribute more to subsequent development of schizophrenia than postnatal exposure. In humans, actual viral infection has not been definitively shown to directly cause schizophrenia in the offspring of infected mothers, but there is increasing evidence that it is a contributing factor. For instance, maternal exposure to HSV-2 has been theorized to cause schizophrenia and schizoaffective disorders. Yet, a study by Alan Brown and colleagues (2006) did not find any support for a relationship between HSV-2 and subsequent schizophrenia and schizoaffective disorder in the offspring of infected mothers. On the other hand, a case-control study did show a significant increased risk for the development of psychoses among offspring of mothers who had been exposed to HSV-2 (Buka et al., 2008). The risk was even greater if the mothers had high rates of sexual activity during their pregnancy.

A study in mice suggests that a disruption of the balance of cytokines in mothers during gestation may lead to neurodevelopmental problems in their offspring (Meyer et al., 2006; Meyer, Murray, et al., 2008; Meyer, Nyffeler, et al., 2008). Another study with rats has shown that malnourishment in mothers is related to pro-inflammatory factors that may increase the risk of schizophrenia among their offspring (J. Xu et al., 2015). S. Hossein Fatemi and colleagues (2008) examined the effects of maternal infection in mice with subsequent effects on brain structure and function. They showed that infection near the end of the second trimester of pregnancy could lead to abnormal gene expression in the brain and subsequent structural defects that could be related to schizophrenia and autism. Vijay Mittal and associates (2008) found that adolescents diagnosed with schizotypal personality disorder who had prenatal exposure to a viral teratogen were at increased risk for developing schizophrenia when compared to a similar group who did not have exposure. They conclude that the risk of psychosis is increased among the offspring of infected mothers. However, they note that mothers of high-risk children tended to over-report exposure to infectious disease.

Autoimmune hypothesis of schizophrenia

In the 1980s, John Knight (1982), proposed that autoantibodies affected neurons in the limbic region of the brain, thereby causing schizophrenia. There is now an increasing amount of evidence that supports the idea that some cases of schizophrenia may originate as an autoimmune process (Severance et al., 2016). A recent study found that the genes responsible for producing the cytokine Interleukin-8 (IL-8) were highly expressed in people suffering from schizophrenia, causing greater production of the cytokine when compared to a control group. The results suggest that IL-8 could be responsible for pathophysiological changes in the brain that occur in people suffering from schizophrenia (L. Xu et al., 2018).

Lending credence to the autoimmune hypothesis of schizophrenia, another study found that the presence of many autoimmune diseases increased the risk of developing schizophrenia. Specifically, people suffering from systemic lupus erythematosus had 3.73 times more risk of developing schizophrenia. People suffering from rheumatoid arthritis had a 2.89 times increase in risk and those with dermatomyositis had 5.85 times the risk of developing schizophrenia respectively. This contradicts reports that did not find an association between arthritis and schizophrenia (Cullen et al., 2019). Autoimmune vasculitis increased risk of developing schizophrenia by 2.44 times. This study also found that steroid use protected against developing schizophrenia (L.-Y. Wang et al., 2018).

Other researchers conducted a meta-analysis of research on the relationship between non-neurological autoimmune (NNAI) disorders and psychoses. They found an overall positive relationship between NNAIs and psychoses. Those with NNAIs were 1.26 times more likely to develop a psychosis. However, the specific disorders differed from the previous study cited above. People suffering from pernicious anemia and those with pemphigoid had 1.9 times greater odds of becoming schizophrenic, while those with psoriasis, celiac disease, and Graves' disease had 1.7, 1.5, and 1.3 times greater odds, respectively, of having schizophrenia. On the other hand, those suffering from ankylosing spondylitis and rheumatoid arthritis had about 0.7 times decreased odds for developing the disorder. It is possible that inflammatory pathways, genetics, autoantibodies targeting brain proteins, and exposure to corticosteroids underlie the observed associations (Cullen et al., 2019).

A study of the connection between the genetics of autoimmune disorders and schizophrenia did not find genetic overlap in common single nucleotide polymorphisms that could explain comorbidity in autoimmune disorders and schizophrenia (Hoeffding et al., 2017). However, as discussed above, polygenic and epigenetic studies have yielded evidence of an association between immunity and schizophrenia. The role of gastrointestinal disorders has been examined as a link between autoimmune disorders and schizophrenia (Severance, Prandovszky, Castiglione, & Yolken, 2015). One hypothesis is that exposure to wheat gluten and bovine milk casein creates gut inflammation and humeral immunity to food antigens, which occur early during the course of schizophrenia. The gut inflammation can increase gut permeability that allows gut bacteria to translocate into the circulatory system. This can trigger innate immunity including activation of C1q, which also functions in brain synapses. T. gondii infection is also known to initiate gut inflammation and could affect activation of immune responses in the brain in the same way. Immigrants, who are known to be at greater risk for schizophrenia, may be forced to modify their diets in a way that promotes gut inflammation and immune system activation affecting the brain. The authors conclude that an understanding of the disrupted microbiome can provide useful models of brain pathogenesis (Severance et al., 2016).

A review by Nadia Cattane and her colleagues (2020) examined research on the relationship of dysbiosis of the human gut microbiota (GMB) and schizophrenia. The GMB produces a number of compounds, including neurotransmitters, which could influence central nervous system functioning. The GMB is thought to be a mediator of pre- and postnatal environmental insults. A number of studies have demonstrated that the GMB of people suffering from neurodevelopmental disorders including schizophrenia differs from non-psychiatric subjects. Stress may play a role in the dysbiosis of the GMB,

> ... several insults, such as inflammatory insults and/or stressful experiences, could modify the GMB composition leading to an imbalance between bacteria with anti-inflammatory and pro-inflammatory properties. An enrichment of bacteria with pro-inflammatory properties causes then a higher gut barrier permeability, which in turn could lead to the passage of both inflammation mediators and bacteria components, including their endotoxins or metabolites, from the gut to the blood circulation and then possibly to the brain. (p. 266)

In early life the composition of the GMB is important for the development of a healthy immune system. Gut dysbiosis at this time could lead to a chronic inflammatory state that could negatively influence brain functioning. The GMB has also been shown to be associated with cognitive impairment in people with serious mental illnesses such as schizophrenia, suggesting gut biota could be used as cognitive enhancers in this population (Bioque et al., 2021). The accumulating research on the relationship of GMB to schizophrenia suggests that better understanding of the role of gut pathogens, the microbiome, and their effects on the brain could lead to immunologic and microbial methods of prevention and treatment (Severance & Yolken, 2020).

CHAPTER 3

Neurobiology of schizophrenia

Much research is focused on the role of neurobiology in schizophrenia. However, the relationship of neurobiology to understanding the causes of the disease is still being debated (Brambilla & Tansella, 2007). While neurobiology is undoubtedly important, it is thought that the etiology of schizophrenia is multifactorial (K. Dean et al., 2003).

The neurotransmitter dopamine has long been suspected as a key component of schizophrenic pathology. The so-called "dopamine hypothesis" of schizophrenia grew from the observation that drugs that increase the activity of dopamine in the brain can also induce psychosis. Conversely drugs that block dopamine receptors were found to reduce psychotic symptoms (Baumeister & Francis, 2002). Briefly, the dopamine hypothesis asserts that in normal people the prefrontal dopamine system controls the limbic dopamine system through suppression. In individuals suffering from schizophrenia the activity of the dopaminergic neurons in the prefrontal dopamine system is reduced causing overactivity of the limbic dopamine system. The reduced activity of the prefrontal dopamine neurons is responsible for the negative symptoms of schizophrenia while the overactivity of the limbic basal ganglia dopamine system is responsible for the positive symptoms of the disease (Gründer & Cumming, 2016; Ohara, 2007).

Some studies have demonstrated increased dopaminergic activity in the mesolimbic pathway of the brain as well as abnormalities in cortical cholinergic transmission in people with schizophrenia (Masciotra et al., 2005; Sarter et al., 2005). Other neurotransmitters may work in concert with dopamine to form the basis of schizophrenic pathology. In normal people the action of dopamine is mediated by receptors on pyramidal and local circuit neurons that stabilize cortical representations of external and internal stimuli. In people with schizophrenia this mediation effect may be reduced, and along with dysfunction in gamma aminobutyric acid (GABA) and glutamate transmission, may contribute to cortical dysfunction (Winterer, 2006).

A number of studies suggest that dysfunction in the neurotransmitter GABA may be important in understanding schizophrenia. Abnormal GABA transmission in the brain may be related to cognitive, affective, sensory, and motor problems in people with schizophrenia. A study assessing expression levels of GABA-related genes in the dorsolateral prefrontal cortex, anterior cingulate cortex (ACC), primary motor cortex, and primary visual cortex found reduced gene expression among subjects suffering from schizophrenia when compared to healthy controls. The authors concluded that since the areas studied represent major functional areas of the cortex, abnormality of GABA transmission may be a contributing factor to a number of different schizophrenic symptoms (Hashimoto et al., 2008). An imaging study using proton magnetic resonance spectroscopy found lower levels of GABA in the ACC and frontal cortex of patients suffering from schizophrenia when compared to healthy control subjects. These differences were especially pronounced in first episode patients with schizophrenia (Kumar et al., 2020).

Some speculation related to the dopamine hypothesis suggests an important role for the N-methyl-D-aspartate (NMDA) receptor for the neurotransmitter glutamate, as these receptors regulate dopamine neurons in the cortex. Inhibition of the functioning of these receptors can bring about both the positive and negative symptoms of schizophrenia. This NMDA receptor hypofunction hypothesis of schizophrenia is supported by the observation that drugs like PCP, which reduce

NMDA function, cause both negative and positive schizophrenic symptoms (Jentsch & Roth, 1999). Nevertheless, there are still issues to be worked out with this approach (Gilmour et al., 2012). There is some evidence that GABA-A receptors are disrupted in patients suffering from schizophrenia. There is some clinical evidence that when benzo-diazepines, which act on GABA-A receptors, are administered with antipsychotic medications, better therapeutic outcomes are achieved than with antipsychotic medication alone (Włodarczyk et al., 2017).

There is an increasing amount of evidence that points to the role of limbic-corticostriatal glutamate transmission pathology as an underlying basis for schizophrenia. A review of the literature by Karen Szumlinski & Todd Kippin (2008) lists six findings that support this theory: smaller cortical volumes, reduced glutamatergic unmyelinated neuronal processes, fewer dendritic spines, pyramidal cell disarray, expression alteration in glutamate receptor subtypes, and reduced expression of cortical synaptic proteins. They go on to explain that the mainstream view is that these glutamate abnormalities in schizophrenia cause hypofrontality, or a reduction in cortical activity and activation. The authors also note that there are other theories that hold the opposite view, in other words that glutamate hyperactivation caused by a disinhibition of glutamate transmission underlies the psychotic and cognitive abnormalities present in schizophrenia.

Serotonin receptor pathology in the cortex has been hypothesized to be associated with schizophrenia and other illnesses such as bipolar disorder. Alteration of serotonin receptors may be subtle and may differ according to gender (Gray et al., 2006). Studies examining the contribution of genetic variation of serotonin-related receptors to schizophrenia have indicated that certain alleles, as well as the synergy among different alleles, may increase susceptibility to schizophrenia (Lorenzo et al., 2006). Serotonin (5-HT) function, which is known to be related to aggressive behavior in general, may also be related to aggressiveness among people suffering from schizophrenia (Barkan et al., 2006).

Other serotonin receptors may play a role in schizophrenia. Brian Dean and his colleagues (2006) have shown that decreased levels of serotonin-sub-7 receptors in Brodmann's area 9 may be related to schizophrenic pathology in a post-mortem study of patients suffering from schizophrenia and in rats. These results are supported by the fact that cortical serotonin-sub-7 and -sub(1D) receptors are affected by antipsychotic drugs among individuals suffering from schizophrenia (Barkan et al., 2006; B. Dean et al., 2001; B. Dean et al., 2006). Additional studies have found that variations in serotonin transport related genes may be associated with increased susceptibility to schizophrenia as well as suicidal behavior among individuals suffering from schizophrenia (De Luca et al., 2006; Fan & Sklar, 2005).

Antipsychotic drugs that are partial agonists to serotonin-5-HT-sub(1A) receptors have improved cognition, including attention, executive function, verbal learning, and memory in some studies with patients suffering from schizophrenia (Sumiyoshi et al., 2007). Other drugs targeting serotonin reuptake inhibition have not been definitively shown to be useful in treating the negative symptoms of schizophrenia. A meta-analysis examining well-designed studies found that the negative symptoms of schizophrenia did not improve when medication was augmented with serotonin reuptake inhibitors. While some studies have shown alterations in the 5HT-sub(1a) receptor binding parameters in schizophrenia patients at post-mortem, a study with living patients did not find any relationship between schizo-phrenic symptoms and 5H-sub(1a) binding (Sepehry et al., 2007). Therefore, there is some question about the role of 5HT-sub(1a) receptors in the pathophysiology of schizophrenia (Frankle et al., 2006). Other studies have not found any association between 5-HT receptor polymorphism and schizophrenia (Kapelski et al., 2006).

CHAPTER 4

Brain structure and schizophrenia

The anterior cingulate cortex (ACC) has been identified as a key area in the pathology of schizophrenia. Most studies of the ACC have focused on fairly simple measurements such as volume when comparing individuals suffering from schizophrenia to normal controls. One study using case control methodology and a novel scanning method was able to show reduced bilateral thickness in the paralimbic region of the ACC along with increased surface area in both the limbic and paralimbic ACC among subjects suffering from schizophrenia. No differences were found in gray matter volume, surface curvature, or central sulcus depth. This study illustrates the rapidly increasing sophistication of brain structure studies of schizophrenia (Fornito et al., 2008).

Limbic system pathology has become one of the focal areas of research in schizophrenia. Limbic areas of the brains in adults suffering from schizophrenia differ consistently from healthy people, but areas outside the limbic system also show differences. Children and adolescents with schizophrenia, however, tend to just have differences in the limbic system as opposed to the whole brain. This has led to the hypothesis that brain pathology associated with schizophrenia starts in the limbic system and then spreads over time. It also may be the case that the limbic pathology is just part of a more global brain abnormality (White et al., 2008).

A number of studies have now shown that people suffering from schizophrenia have both anatomical and functional brain-wide connection dysfunction when compared to healthy people. These dysfunctions are thought to be the main mechanism for the pathophysiology of schizophrenia (Wotruba et al., 2014). One study found a decrease in the connections within and between limbic structures. There was also observed reduction in fibers connecting to the left fronto-temporal region in people suffering from schizophrenia when compared to healthy subjects. This is thought to be evidence for the fronto-temporal dysconnectivity hypotheses of the pathogenesis of schizophrenia (Ottet et al., 2013).

Research using functional magnetic resonance imaging (fMRI) has been used to compare resting state effective connectivity (rsEC) and resting state functional connectivity (rsFC) in people suffering from schizophrenia with healthy control subjects. Seventeen disruptions in rsEC were found in patients suffering from schizophrenia. These rsEC disruptions were associated with the thalamus and pathways from the limbic areas (including the hippocampus, parahippocampus, and cingulate cortex) to the thalamus. Among patients suffering from schizophrenia rsFC abnormality was found to be distributed throughout the whole brain. Since rsEC provides information about the directionality of connections in the brain, the idea that schizophrenia can be characterized by disruptions in the limbic areas that spread to the thalamus is not far-fetched. It should be possible to use rsEC and rsFC patterns in combination as diagnostic markers for schizophrenia (Hua et al., 2020).

A recent systematic review of the research literature by Judith Gault and her coworkers (2018) provides much evidence that schizophrenia is caused by problems in the dopaminergic circuitry in the brain. The dopamine D receptor gene (DRD2) that exists in the highest quantities in the striatum, is part of the reward circuitry. Abnormalities related to the reward circuit have been associated with schizophrenia. Blockage of the DRD2 receptors by antipsychotic medication has been shown to normalize the reward circuitry and reduce schizophrenic symptoms. Because of the high concentrations of DRD2 in the striatum these areas of the brain could be targets for therapies that seek to normalize striatal dopaminergic circuitry. Also, abnormality in circuitry between the striatum and frontal and temporal lobes of the brain may contribute to negative and cognitive symptoms of schizophrenia. Structures that provide input to the striatum including the ventral tegmental area and hippocampus, as well as structures receiving signals from the striatum such as the basal ganglia, may also contribute to dopamine circuitry pathology. According to the research literature, seven models of schizophrenia related dysfunction based on the above circuit abnormalities are hypothesized. These models suggest that intervention sites for new treatment technologies like deep brain stimulation (DBS) may be found.

CHAPTER 5

Cognition and schizophrenia

Cognitive impairment is a key feature among people suffering from schizophrenia. In general, studies of cognition among people suffering from schizophrenia can be conceptualized into two areas, nonsocial and social cognition. Nonsocial cognition includes processing speed, verbal and visuospatial learning and memory, working memory, attention/vigilance, and reasoning/problem solving. People suffering from schizophrenia demonstrate impairments in all of these cognitive domains as well as having impairments in perception. Studies of people with schizophrenia have shown that patterns of cognitive impairment in schizophrenia differ from other disorders such as dementia and bipolar disorders. The cognitive impairments that accompany schizophrenic illness have negative effects on how well people suffering from schizophrenia are able to function.

Diminished functionality among people suffering from schizophrenia includes the ability to take care of themselves, to work and hold down a job, and the ability to acquire important skills related to rehabilitation (M. F. Green et al., 2019). Antipsychotic medication is known to induce cognitive decline as well as other side effects related to greater morbidity and mortality (Agbeli, 2020). Erin Moran and colleagues (2020) compared cognitive performance among individuals with schizophrenia who were taking antipsychotic medication and not taking antipsychotic medication, with healthy subjects. Given the role of dopamine in reinforcement-based learning it was thought antipsychotic medication might be responsible for some cognitive deficit. The study found that both medicated and non-medicated subjects suffering from schizophrenia had pervasive cognitive deficits when compared to healthy subjects. Deficits were found in reinforcement learning, processing speed, cognitive control, working memory, verbal learning, and relational encoding and retrieval. This study demonstrates that cognitive deficits are attributable primarily to schizophrenic disease and not antipsychotic medication.

However, a study by Nikolai Albert and associates (2019) found that patients suffering from schizophrenia who discontinued antipsychotic medication had better cognitive functioning that those who did not stop taking antipsychotic medication. A study by Susie Fu and her coworkers (2019) also demonstrated that people suffering from schizophrenia who discontinued antipsychotic medication because of negative side effects had improved cognition. Many of these patients were then able to use active coping mechanisms to maintain their recovery. It may be that some patients suffering from schizophrenia have differing cognitive responses to antipsychotic medication depending on their genotype (Nelson et al., 2018).

It is likely that there are overlapping biological pathways in schizophrenia and normal cognitive ability. Genes associated with cognitive performance have been found to be related to genes associated with increased risk of schizophrenic disease. These genes play a role in neurotransmitter systems that are important to cognitive performance (Koch et al., 2020).

It may be the case that cognitive impairment in childhood can be predictive of later development of schizophrenic illness (Dickson et al., 2020). This is important because early identification of schizophrenic risk could help identify those who might benefit from interventions to improve cognitive abilities. Psychoeducational and therapeutic interventions have been shown to lessen the impact of cognitive impairment in people suffering from schizophrenia. It is not known if these interventions work on the social and functional impairments that result from cognitive impairment or whether the techniques work directly to improve cognitive impairment itself. Regardless, psychoeducational and therapeutic interventions have been shown to improve the quality of life for people suffering from schizophrenia (Maurel et al., 2011).

Sleep disorders are common among people who suffer from schizophrenia. Jannicke Laskemoen and associates (2020) found sleep disturbances among people with schizophrenia were related to cognitive impairment. Processing speed and inhibition, which are related to insomnia and hypersomnia, were associated with cognitive impairment in patients suffering from schizophrenia. This suggests that treating sleep disturbances may help cognitive functioning in people suffering from schizophrenia.

CHAPTER 6

Social-cognitive and emotional recognition impairment in schizophrenia

Jonathan Burns (2007) in his book *The Descent of Madness* presents an argument that schizophrenia is the by-product of the evolution of the human brain. The same genes that evolved to give humans a highly social brain are also responsible for the potential development of schizophrenia in our species. Enhanced social-cognitive skills gave early humans a huge fitness advantage and were therefore selected for during evolution even though, for a small percentage of the population, this genetic gift could go awry and cause schizophrenia. The ability to read emotional states in others is an important social-cognitive skill that has survival value for humans. Individuals suffering from schizophrenia are known to have difficulty in reading emotions in others, especially facial affect (Kee et al., 2006).

A study by Raquel Gur and her associates (2007) demonstrated that when patients diagnosed with schizophrenia performed an emotional identification task, they showed reduced activation of the limbic system compared to healthy controls. For healthy people correct identification of threat-related facial expressions was associated with increased amygdala activation. Patients suffering from schizophrenia reacted just the opposite, showing decreased activation of the amygdala when confronted with threat expressions. When presented with fearful faces subjects suffering from schizophrenia responded with increased amygdala activation, but with a flat affect. The authors theorized this reaction might be related to overstimulation of the limbic system. They concluded that the abnormal activation of the amygdala in response to threat and fearful facial expression could lead to misidentification of emotions in others.

Another study examined subjects suffering from schizophrenia and normal subjects while they engaged in tasks involving intuitive and cognitive emotional conditions. When subjects suffering from schizophrenia performed the emotional recognition tasks the limbic areas of the brain related to processing of emotions failed to activate. Subjects suffering from schizophrenia showed reduced activation in areas of the brain related to holistic processing of facial features and instead showed increased activity in brain regions that analyze facial features. The results suggest that subjects suffering from schizophrenia lack the ability to intuitively read affect in others and compensate for this loss by using a more cognitive approach to identifying features related to emotions in others (Fakra et al., 2008).

An additional study examining gaze discrimination impairment found that subjects suffering from schizophrenia and healthy control subjects have similar gaze discrimination abilities. Yet the people suffering from schizophrenia showed reduced brain activity in areas related to executive, emotional, and visual processing. When performing more difficult tasks, the healthy control subjects showed increased activation in the frontal and temporal regions of the brain. Increased activation was found in people suffering from schizophrenia when they were directly gazing at another face. The authors concluded that the results may be related to the problems people with schizophrenia have in interacting with other people (Kohler et al., 2008).

A study examining the disconnection of the autonomic arousal in the amygdala related to fear found individuals suffering from schizophrenia had abnormally increased arousal along with reductions in emotion-specific regions and the medial prefrontal cortex. The authors concluded that when confronted with signals for danger the central and autonomic processing in people suffering from schizophrenia is disconnected. This type of dysfunction might be related to paranoid symptoms such as delusions (Williams et al., 2007). Some of this dysfunction could be related to suboptimal parental bonding in people suffering from schizophrenia. As mentioned above, people suffering from schizophrenia are more likely to have experienced childhood trauma and to have impairments in parental bonding and social cognitive skills. Physical neglect was found to be especially predictive of impairment in emotional recognition. However, optimal parental bonding attenuated the negative impact of childhood trauma on emotional recognition (Rokita et al., 2020).

CHAPTER 7

Treatment of schizophrenia

Historically, schizophrenia has been treated with a wide variety of modalities that were not especially effective. Trepanation, exorcism, beating, spinning, and hydrotherapy (immersion in both hot and cold water) were some of the early treatments for schizophrenia (Braslow, 1999; González de Chávez, 2009; Høyersten, 1996; Whitaker, 2002). Treatments such as immersion in water continued well into the modern era and could be brutal and dangerous. One of the authors of this book (K. Volkan) is a founder of a university housed at the site of a former mental hospital. When he first arrived at his job, he was directed to go to an old hospital building that was being used as a warehouse where office furniture was being stored. There among the desks and chairs was a hydrotherapy apparatus that had been used with patients suffering from schizophrenia, presumably until the hospital closed down in the late 1990s.

Physical torment, especially in the form of beatings, has dogged people suffering from schizophrenia throughout history (Whitaker, 2002). Like hydrotherapy, beating has only lately gone out of style even though it has long been outlawed. Beating was not so much a treatment but a form of patient management. Other forms of violence served as ways to manage patients into compliance while masquerading as treatments.

Neuromodulation

By the late nineteenth and early twentieth centuries new treatments were being invented to treat schizophrenia and other severe mental illnesses. Primitive neuromodulation treatments in the form of convulsive therapies using insulin, Cardiazol, Metrazol, and eventually electricity became routine for people suffering from schizophrenia. These forms of convulsive therapies were considered to reduce psychotic symptoms. Electroshock (ECT) became the preferred method because it was cheap and thought to be less dangerous than the other methods. ECT was thought to work by damaging the brain, causing the stripping away of the intellect. Psychotic symptoms were abated but this was short-lived, requiring further sessions and further damage to the brain. ECT could be especially dangerous when multiple sessions were administered over a short period of time. Strong muscle convulsions also caused bone breakage in up to 40% of patients (Whitaker, 2002).

In his book, *Large-Group Psychology: Racism, Societal Divisions, Narcissistic Leaders and Who We Are Now*, Vamık Volkan (2020) writes about seeing African American patients at Cherry Hospital in Goldsboro, North Carolina in the early 1960s. After coming to the USA in 1957, and after completing his psychiatric training at the University of North Carolina at Chapel Hill he was assigned to Cherry Hospital in Goldsboro, North Carolina as a new psychiatrist. When this hospital was opened in August 1880 its name was "Asylum for Colored Insane." It was one of the first mental hospitals designated only for African Americans. In the early 1960s, Cherry Hospital was still only for African American individuals. Vamık Volkan recalls that there was not a single white physician working at this hospital who was born in the United States. The care of African American mental patients was given completely to immigrant white doctors. He describes his experience of seeing the Cherry Hospital patients receiving ECT:

> In those days there was a morning routine at Cherry Hospital. About 100 patients would receive electric shock therapy. The patients would line up two by two and wait to enter the room where they were restrained on a stretcher. Wires would be attached to their forehead and an attendant would put a piece of cloth in their mouth in order to prevent them from biting their tongue while

convulsing. No anesthetics were given. A white doctor would push a button to produce the electricity. I, too, was "ordered" to give electric shock therapy; otherwise, I would lose my job. One day I clearly associated the line of patients waiting to be electrically shocked with lines of Jewish people I had seen in films being guided to gas chambers. I felt shame and guilt. (p. 74)

There was no research at Cherry Hospital to illustrate if electric shock therapy was helping patients suffering from schizophrenia and it certainly did not help patients who had been essentially incarcerated in a mental hospital due to their race.

The other author of this book, Kevin Volkan worked in a locked-in facility with a number of patients in California that had been diagnosed with schizophrenia and who suffered from the consequences of intensive electroshock treatment. Here is his description of one older Asian gentleman:

Huang had been committed to a mental hospital in the late 1930s and diagnosed schizophrenia. Nevertheless, he did not appear psychotic. Digging through his hospital records I discovered that as a young man in his 20s Huang had been committed for "rowdy behavior and getting into fights." The Chinese Exclusion Act, which was passed in 1882 and not repealed until 1943, reflected the discriminatory attitude towards Asians that was prevalent at the time and offered an explanation why a young Chinese man could be sent against his will to a mental hospital for infractions that would have earned mild penalties for a white person. Once in the mental hospital, Huang was subjected to the typical routine prescribed for patients diagnosed with schizophrenia at that time and was given a course of ECT that consisted of multiple sessions per week extending over 2 months. This course of ECT treatment left Huang with brain damage. Afterwards he had trouble reading and speaking clearly, as well as with issues with motor functions. It seems that even after the ECT treatment Huang was thought to require further treatment and a little while later he was given a lobotomy. When I worked with him in the late 1970s Huang was a friendly person who very much liked to show that he could read. In a stuttering and halting voice, Huang would read out loud from the newspaper, proudly displaying this ability with a degree of self-satisfaction, before shuffling back to his room where he spent most of the day. Huang never demonstrated any signs of schizophrenia during my time with him, but still carried the diagnosis. At that time Huang had lived in mental hospitals for around 40 years and was destined to spend the rest of his life in this environment.

While ECT is now not often used in psychiatry it has become much safer with the concurrent administration of muscle relaxants, lower current, and the use of ultra-brief pulsed stimulation that is not thought to cause permanent brain damage. Modern ECT is mostly used to treat pharmacoresistant mood disorders but has been used to treat schizophrenia as well. ECT is also used to treat schizophrenia in parts of the world where antipsychotics are not practical for financial reasons (Gazdag & Ungvari, 2019).

There are positive anecdotal reports as to the clinical effectiveness of treating schizophrenia with modern ECT though large studies are lacking (Rado & Hernandez, 2014). Research evidence is emerging for the effectiveness of modern ECT in treating pharmacoresistant schizophrenia. A small study by Philipp Thomann and his colleagues (2017) used modern ECT with pharmacoresistant patients suffering from schizophrenia and major depressive disorder (MDD) to research changes in brain structure and function. Right-sided unilateral ECT was found to change brain structure and function regardless of diagnosis. All patients in the study experienced improvement in their clinical symptoms. Seven patients suffering from MDD achieved remission and the other four experienced at least a 50% improvement. Four patients suffering from schizophrenia experienced at least a 50% improvement while the other five subjects experienced 25% improvement at minimum.

Other non-invasive methods of neuromodulation have been developed in recent years, but they are primarily used for treating mood disorders and are not thought to be as effective as modern ECT:

> Additional non-invasive therapies include magnetic seizure therapy, which focally induces the superficial cortex to produce seizures, repetitive transcranial magnetic stimulation, involving the pulse application of magnetic stimuli to alter cortical excitability, and vagal nerve stimulation, which sends electrical impulses

to various brain regions via the solitary nucleus … The role for these alternative treatments remains unclear, as ECT is generally considered clinically superior. (Staudt et al., 2019, p. 4)

Nevertheless, Emmanuel Poulet and associates (2008) report that the use of transcranial magnetic stimulation (TMS) reduced resistant auditory hallucinations. A study by Flavio Fröhlich and Caroline Lustenberger (2020) speculates that non-invasive neuromodulation may be able to correct sleep abnormalities among people suffering from schizophrenia. Jeffrey Rado and Edgar Hernandez (2014) report that TMS combined with a small amount of electric current shows promise in treating schizophrenia.

Psychosurgery

Beside convulsive therapies, the other treatment that was widely used to treat schizophrenia was psychosurgery. Michael Staudt and colleagues (2019) have given an excellent review of the history of psychosurgery and the section below is mostly drawn from their work. Gottlieb Burckhardt first reported performing the excision of regions of the brain with six patients in 1888. After being inspired by research on the removal of the frontal lobes in primates, Portuguese physicians Edgar Moniz and neurosurgeon Almeida Lima developed a procedure for creating lesions in the frontal lobes called a leucotomy. This was used to treat depression, anxiety, and aggression.

In the United States the neurologist–neurosurgeon team of Walter Freeman and James Watts refined Moniz's procedure and renamed it the prefrontal lobotomy. A minimal form of the procedure was used for patients with affective disorders while a more invasive radical form was used for people suffering from schizophrenia. Freeman later adopted the technique of transorbital lobotomy that was developed by Italian psychiatrist Amarro Fiamberti. This technique involved sedating the patient with ECT, inserting an "ice pick-like" instrument through the orbital socket, and performing sweeping motions to destroy areas of the frontal lobes of the brain. This operation could be done by minimally trained physicians without the need for a surgeon or anesthesiologist and without the need for a specialized operating theater.

Freeman ambitiously advocated for the technique and it became quite popular. Transorbital lobotomies were performed throughout America and Europe. It is estimated that Freeman himself performed over 3000 procedures from the 1930s through the 1960s, with tens of thousands performed around the world (Caruso & Sheehan, 2017). Freeman claimed almost miraculous results from transorbital lobotomies, but as in many of the early treatments what counted as success was highly questionable and biased by the lack of scientific study. Some of Freeman's patients claimed long-term improvement but this was not the majority. It is likely that patients had a very different view about what was considered a cure or improvement than many mental health professionals. For the latter, a positive outcome was anything that made patients easier to manage. The book *One Flew Over the Cuckoo's Nest* (Kesey, 1962) and subsequent film (Forman, 1975) dramatically illustrate this.

Freeman performed his last transorbital lobotomy in 1967 on a patient that had twice previously had the procedure. Unfortunately, he nicked a blood vessel and the patient died. Shortly thereafter, Freeman retired from practice and drove around the country in his recreational vehicle interviewing former patients about their positive experience with the operation. It is interesting to note that over time Freeman relaxed the indications for the transorbital lobotomy. He increasingly saw it as a panacea and by the end of his career he was lobotomizing children. In one notable case he lobotomized Howard Dully, a twelve-year-old boy who was having problems adjusting to the death of his mother and getting along with his stepmother (Dully & Fleming, 2007). Many physicians were not enthusiastic about transorbital lobotomies and when the first antipsychotic medication, chlorpromazine (trade name Thorazine) became available (and marketed as a lobotomy in a bottle) it was enthusiastically adopted as the primary treatment for schizophrenia (López-Muñoz et al., 2005).

More precise forms of psychosurgery are still performed in very few cases but are mostly used to treat obsessive-compulsive disorder (Brakoulias et al., 2019). Nevertheless, the idea of using psychosurgery to treat schizophrenia has recently reemerged, albeit in far more subtle and less invasive forms. Deep brain stimulation (DBS) that involves placing an electrode that can deliver a small amount of current directly into the brain is now being proposed as a treatment for schizophrenia. In one study DBS was shown to prevent the emergence of sensorimotor gating, attentional selectivity, and executive functioning deficits in a rat model of schizophrenia (Hadar et al., 2018).

Judith Gault and her associates (2018) review the growing interest in using neuromodulation via DBS to treat schizophrenia. As mentioned previously, they report on seven models of predominantly striatal dysregulation that provide possible therapeutic targets. The authors report that DBS could be used to correct dysregulation in these target circuits as well as treat areas of the brain related to tardive dyskinesia (a side effect from antipsychotic medication) and negative and cognitive symptoms of schizophrenia. In two research reviews where DBS was used in the ventral cortex and ventral striatum, the following reports were highlighted.

The first report was a patient who suffered from obsessive compulsive disorder, which is characterized by the uncontrollable repetition of thoughts and behaviors (OCD), and residual schizophrenic symptoms. While the negative symptoms of schizophrenia did not change for this patient, their OCD symptoms and psychosocial functioning improved 25%–58%.

The second patient who suffered from schizophrenia was part of a clinical trial using DBS to alleviate symptoms in treatment-resistant schizophrenia. This study used a protocol with patients randomized to receive DBS at either the medial prefrontal cortex or nucleus accumbens. DBS stimulation would then remain on for three months, after which responsive patients would be crossed over to either a stimulation on or stimulation off group. This was a small trial of eight planned patients. The one patient to finish the trial demonstrated a 62% reduction in positive symptoms and a 33% improvement in negative symptoms. This patient initially received bilateral stimulation after adjusting to unilateral left sided stimulation. However, bilateral stimulation caused akathisia and the patient was returned to unilateral stimulation that resulted in a relapse of negative symptoms. Positive symptoms remained improved.

Another trial is slated to target the pars reticulata of the substantia nigra in order to modulate activity in the basal ganglia, as well as the medial dorsal and lateral prefrontal cortex. This is hypothesized to normalize medial dorsal activity and improve both cognitive and positive symptoms of schizophrenia. Lastly, a trial that was to use DBS targeting the ventral striatum and ventral tegmental area closed due to an inability to enroll patients.

A prospective, non-control group study treated schizophrenia with capsulotomy. This therapy, which has been used for severe cases of treatment-resistant OCD, involves the bilateral destruction of brain tissue in the internal capsule. The study reported improvement in 74% of patients suffering from schizophrenia. Capsulotomy has been used for a number of years for people suffering with treatment resistant OCD. In one study of nineteen severe OCD patients receiving capsulotomy seven of them fully responded to the surgery (meaning their OCD scores improved by at least 35%), while 10% had a partial response (i.e. their OCD scores improved by 25%). Three patients achieved remission. More than half the patients did not respond. These patients had suffered severe OCD for a longer time. Capsulotomy is not without risk. Two patients in the study suffered permanent complications including paralysis and cognitive impairment (D'Astous et al., 2013). Given the limited success rate and risk of capsulotomy, DBS, which is thought to be just as effective, may be a more promising treatment.

In their review Judith Gault and her associates (2018) argue that people suffering from schizophrenia should have access to the possible benefits of DBS, but also caution that patients suffering from severe schizophrenia may not have the capacity to consent to such an invasive procedure.

Antipsychotic medication

Since the 1950s schizophrenia has been generally treated with a variety of antipsychotic medications that alleviate the symptoms of the disease, but not the underlying pathology. Most of these drugs work by suppressing dopamine activity in the brain, and because of this, have many serious side effects such as tardive dyskinesia (Baumeister & Francis, 2002). While newer antipsychotic medications also affect the function of other neurotransmitters (B. Dean et al., 2006; Hagiwara et al., 2008), dopamine targets still play a key role in the newer drugs that treat schizophrenia (Seeman, 2000). The fact that newer second-generation antipsychotic drugs do not seem to be more effective than first generation antipsychotic drugs supports the importance of dopamine as a target for medication (Lewis & Lieberman, 2008; J. A. Lieberman et al., 2005). Unfortunately, second generation antipsychotic medications also retain many of the side effects of the first generation drugs (Divac et al., 2014). Nevertheless, dopamine agonist antipsychotic medications have the best evidence for effectiveness in treating the symptoms of schizophrenia (Tandon et al., 2010).

While treatment with antipsychotic drugs has been in existence for almost seventy years, there are still many important unanswered questions related to using them to treat individuals with schizophrenic and other psychotic disorders. Questions related to choice of drug, dosage, when and if another drug should be tried, monitoring the effects of the drug treatment, and whether drugs can halt or slow the progression of the illness remain without definitive answers. While medicine in general has been moving towards "evidence based" treatment, the treatment of people suffering from schizophrenia largely remains precedent and experientially based—that is, based on what an individual physician was taught and what they intuit to be best for a given patient (Davis & Leucht, 2008; Kane & Leucht, 2008).

Many people who suffer from schizophrenia may need to be hospitalized at some time in their lives. Hospitalization allows the patient to stabilize and receive regular doses of medication and is generally short in duration. However, when medication compliance is poor, patients suffering from schizophrenia may destabilize once they leave the inpatient setting and require re-hospitalization. This creates a "revolving door" through the mental health system. A recent study supports this view, demonstrating that patients suffering from schizophrenia who take their antipsychotic medication on a regular basis have fewer and shorter incidences of hospitalization (dosReis et al., 2008).

Likewise, non-adherence to a medication regime has been shown to increase the risk of relapse after a first psychotic episode (Alvarez-Jimenez et al., 2012). Another study concluded that not treating first episode psychosis with antipsychotic medication may lead to increased brain pathogenesis (Kraguljac et al., 2020). Yet there have been some studies that question the use of antipsychotic medication in first episode psychosis. A Finnish study found that patients suffering from first episode schizophrenia who were given minimal antipsychotic medication along with treatment that included intensive psychosocial intervention did as well or even better than patients treated with typical heavy use of antipsychotic drugs (Lehtinen et al., 2000). Another study of first episode psychosis found that 41% of patients who refused antipsychotic medication achieved symptomatic remission with 33% achieving functional recovery. Predictors of symptomatic remission included better pre-morbid functioning, higher education level, and being employed. Functional recovery was related to less severe psychopathology, shorter duration of prodromal phase, and less use of cannabis (Conus et al., 2017). As we shall see later, these findings could be important in determining which individuals who suffer from schizophrenia may be amenable to psychotherapeutic intervention.

Most currently available antipsychotic medications are primarily effective against the positive symptoms of schizophrenia. Negative and cognitive symptoms have been more difficult to treat. So-called second generation or atypical antipsychotic drugs have not proven to be more effective than first generation antipsychotic medications in dealing with these symptoms (J. A. Lieberman et al., 2005). It may even be the case that first generation antipsychotic drugs are superior to second generation antipsychotics (Foussias & Remington, 2010).

A review by Amanda Krogmann, and colleagues (2019) outlines a number of mono- and add-on therapeutic agents that are now being examined for their ability to treat schizophrenia. Some of these drugs are targeted towards positive and negative symptoms, negative symptoms alone, and residual and treatment-resistant positive symptoms. These drugs include dopamine receptor 1, 2, and 3 (D1, D2, D3) agonists, 5-hydroxytryptamine (serotonin) receptor (5HT) agonists and inhibiters, a dopamine receptor 1-regulated NMDA (glutamate) receptor and α-amino-3-hydroxy-5-methyl-4-isoxazolepropionic acid (glutamate) receptor (AMPA) agonists, phosphodiesterase 10A enzyme (PDE10A) inhibitors, trace amine-associated receptor 1 (TAAR1) agonists, a nitric oxide donor, a sigma2 receptor (which is highly expressed in malignant cancer cells) antagonist, an alpha1-adrenergic (which is involved in norepinephrine and epinephrine signaling) antagonist, and a D-amino acid oxidase (DAAO—which produces ammonia and hydrogen peroxide affecting the brain) inhibitor. In addition, a number of existing antipsychotic drugs have been reformulated into long-lasting and injectable formulations to improve adherence to antipsychotic medication regimens. Lastly a μ-opioid receptor antagonist is being tested to reduce Olanzapine-induced weight gain, associated cardiovascular issues, and (one assumes) constipation. The clinical trial results for these new therapeutic agents have been mixed. While progress has been made, challenges remain in finding a balance between side effects and adherence to the medication regimen for dopamine modulating medications. With regard to non-dopamine modulating novel drugs, the authors state:

> These studies will need to prove that, in fact, such non-dopamine modulating agents can improve negative symptoms while maintaining positive symptom stability, despite the removal of the prior dopamine modulating antipsychotic agent that at one point was needed to reduce schizophrenia symptoms. (p. 63)

They conclude that despite an urgent need for better pharmacological agents to treat schizophrenia, these will likely not be forthcoming until the pathophysiology of the disease is better understood.

Anti-inflammatory and immunomodulating agents

As described above, immunity, autoimmunity, and inflammation may play a role in schizophrenia. The evidence linking autoimmune disorders and schizophrenia suggests that immunosuppressive therapies might be helpful in treating schizophrenia (Chaudhry et al., 2015; Knight et al., 2007). However, immunosuppressive therapies have had mixed results. It does seem that at least some cases of schizophrenia have an immunological component and that prevention of immune triggers may be helpful for high-risk populations (Richard & Brahm, 2012). Evidence exists indicating there are abnormalities in cell-mediated processed, acute phase proteins, cytokines, and intracellular mediators among people suffering from schizophrenia. One study found that pro-inflammatory cytokines are increased in the blood of patients suffering from schizophrenia. Antipsychotic medication was not found to be a confounding factor (B. Miller et al., 2011). C-reactive protein (CRP) may be a marker for low-grade neuroinflammation that can become chronic, damaging the microvascular system in the brain and reducing cerebral blood flow (Singh & Chaudhuri, 2014).

Maternal immune activation can lead to prenatal exposure of pro-inflammatory cytokines, which can in turn cause both acute and long-term changes in neurobehavioral development. These present possible prenatal targets for reducing susceptibility for developing schizophrenia. Treatment targets include neuroprotection and functional enhancement to prevent abnormal structural and functional changes in the brain, reduction of oxidative stress and toxicity, reduction of pro-inflammatory cytokines, increase in anti-inflammatory cytokines, modulation of microglia function, and reduction of environmental stressors (Hong & Bang, 2020).

New treatments based on immunosuppression, immunomodulation, and neuroinflammation are theoretically promising but have not yet been proven. Medications or substances that have anti-inflammatory, immunomodulation, or neuroprotective effects could be repurposed. These include davunetide (an eight amino acid peptide with neuro-protective qualities), IFN-γ-1b (an interferon used to treat multiple sclerosis), mesenchymal stem cells (which can change microglia from an activated to an anti-inflammatory state), minocycline (an antibiotic with anti-inflammatory effects), monoclonal antibodies (which have anti-inflammatory effects), non-steroidal anti-inflammatory drugs (NSAIDS), Omega-3 fatty acids (which have anti-inflammatory effects), and statins (which have anti-inflammatory effects). Other substances could include antioxidant supplements like N-acetylcysteine (which may be neuroprotective), herbal substances such as cannabidiol (the anti-inflammatory non-THC component of the cannabis plant), and foods thought to reduce inflammation. It is possible these could be used in combination and in conjunction with standard pharmacotherapies. It is also possible that optimal use of antipsychotic medication could help reduce inflammation.

However, a potential problem is that antipsychotic medication can cause global immunosuppression. While this effect could enhance the therapeutic effect of the medication for schizophrenia, it could make subjects suffering from schizophrenia more susceptible to diseases and complications related to further immune suppression (May, 1968; Pang et al., 2017).

Also, targeting immune and anti-inflammatory therapies to specific biomarkers and specific clinical subgroups could provide a more personalized, and hopefully, more effective approach to treating schizophrenia (Hong & Bang, 2020; Krogmann et al., 2019; Pandurangi & Buckley, 2020; Sommer et al., 2012).

The role of immunity in the development of schizophrenia continues to be a promising area of research not only for treating schizophrenia but also for its prevention (Dickerson et al., 2017). If a microbial trigger could be found for schizophrenia, it is possible that a vaccine could be developed against the trigger, thereby preventing the disease (Adams et al., 2012). Clearly, more research on the relationship between immunity, schizophrenia, and immunity-mediating treatments needs to be done.

Non-Western and novel treatments for schizophrenia

Research on traditional Chinese medicine suggests that Chinese herbal medicine may work well in combination with antipsychotic drugs (Rathbone et al., 2007). Patients receiving electroacupuncture along with electroconvulsive therapies were shown to have fewer schizophrenic symptoms than controls. In addition, patients receiving electroacupuncture showed reduced weight as well as reduction in headaches, insomnia, dry mouth, and electrocardiographic abnormalities (Jia et al., 2019).

In a review of a number of small studies traditional Indian Ayurvedic medicine showed promise for treating schizophrenia but was not as effective as chlorpromazine in acutely ill people (Agarwal et al., 2007). It has been speculated that Ayurvedic medicine, which has traditionally been used to treat immunologic disorders, may have a positive effect on schizophrenia by acting on the immune system (Juckel & Hoffmann, 2018). An Ayurvedic polyherbal formulation called *brahmi vati* was found to have anticonvulsant and memory enhancement properties, and to counter amphetamine-induced schizophrenia in mice. Brahmi vati has been used since ancient times to treat seizures and schizophrenic symptoms in India (Mishra et al., 2018).

Some studies have indicated that the brains of people suffering from schizophrenia have reduced levels of Omega-3 fatty acids and some think that this may explain the reduced dopamine activity of the prefrontal cortex as well as suggesting Omega-3 fatty acid supplementation as a possible treatment (Ohara, 2007). It may be possible that a subset of patients suffering from schizophrenia can benefit from niacin augmentation (X. J. Xu & Jiang, 2015). Exercise has been shown to improve both positive and negative symptoms of schizophrenia, as well as quality of life, hippocampal function and volume, and cognition (Girdler et al., 2019; Mitsadali et al., 2020; Sabe et al., 2020; Shimada et al., 2019).

CHAPTER 8

Non-psychodynamic therapeutic approaches to treating schizophrenia

Supportive psychotherapy, which includes advising, behavioral reinforcement and shaping, bolstering of defenses, comforting, listening, problem-solving, and reassuring is often offered to people with schizophrenia; however, this is usually to help patients cope with the disease rather than treating the disease itself. A review found that supportive therapy was not any better than standard care and less helpful than a variety of psychotherapeutic approaches with regard to hospitalization, general mental state, and satisfaction with care (Buckley & Pettit, 2007). However, supportive care in a group setting has been shown to be useful (Nightingale & McQueeney, 1996).

There is growing use of cognitive-behavioral therapy (CBT) with patients suffering from schizophrenia. This use of CBT is usually done in concert with the use of antipsychotic medication and has demonstrated a general reduction in symptoms with especially good results in reducing positive and residual symptoms and strengthening reality testing. Depression is also seen as amenable to treatment using CBT among people suffering from schizophrenia (Sudak, 2004; Turkington et al., 2004; Turkington et al., 2003; Warman & Beck, 2003). CBT group therapy has also been tried with patients suffering from schizophrenia. Some studies have shown improvements in overcoming social phobia and depression, but the results are not definitive (Lawrence et al., 2006).

Another study demonstrated a reduction in feelings of hopelessness and low self-esteem using CBT in a group setting with patients suffering from schizophrenia (Barrowclough et al., 2006). In a study of a single patient who suffered from schizophrenia and pathological gambling, CBT combined with medication awareness training was found to reduce the severity of psychotic and pathological gambling symptoms, as well as to improve psychosocial functioning and dispositional mindfulness (Shonin et al., 2014). A study of sixteen patients suffering from schizophrenia spectrum disorders examined the effects of a form of CBT that was manualized and adapted to psychotic patients. The researchers found a reduction of delusional symptoms as well as a decrease in depressive symptoms (Lamster et al., 2018). The effects of CBT tailored to treat insomnia was examined among patients suffering from schizophrenia and insomnia. This study examined three types of insomnia in patients suffering from schizophrenia: classic severe insomnia, insomnia with normal sleep duration, and insomnia with hypersomnia. Patients with classic severe insomnia showed marked improvement in total sleep time while patients suffering from schizophrenia with insomnia and hypersomnia showed reductions in total sleep time. Patients suffering from schizophrenia with insomnia but with normal sleep duration had a blunted response to CBT (Chiu et al., 2018).

Sameer Jauhur and colleagues (2014) conducted a meta-analysis of the effectiveness of CBT for people suffering from schizophrenia. This study pooled data from randomized trials, controlling for randomization, masking of outcomes, incompleteness of data, use of a control, and publication bias. Results demonstrated that the therapeutic effect of CBT is small. In a comment on this study Christian Gold (2015) notes that the data do not show much relationship between positive therapeutic outcomes and the number of sessions. He even suggests that there may be an inverse relationship with better outcomes coming from fewer sessions. Meta-analytic studies are especially helpful because many CBT studies have small numbers and data pooled from multiple studies may provide better estimates of the effectiveness of CBT. In his book *CBT for Schizophrenia: Evidence-based Interventions and Future Directions* Craig Steel (2013) gives an overview of CBT-based treatments that are likely to be helpful to people suffering from schizophrenia. He also makes the case for using specialized CBT protocols that are tailored to specific symptoms such as command hallucinations, violent behavior, and PTSD.

CHAPTER 9

Recovery from schizophrenia

Before the advent of antipsychotic medication most people suffering from schizophrenia in the Western world were relegated to living in institutions or some type of asylum. With the advent of antipsychotic medication, it became possible for people suffering from schizophrenia to exert some control over their psychotic symptoms. However, treatment goals for people suffering from schizophrenia have moved beyond control over symptoms to regaining social and cognitive function and a better quality of life (Silva & Restrepo, 2019).

Hope and self-esteem have been found to contribute to the subjective sense of recovery among people suffering from schizophrenia, suggesting that these should be promoted during recovery (İpçi et al., 2020). One dimension of recovery from schizophrenia is the feeling of not being dominated by psychotic symptoms. This feeling was found to be associated with time spent in self-directed and sustained exercise (Gonzalez-Flores, 2020). In a qualitative study of people suffering from schizophrenia subjects describe facing considerable challenges in functioning but also describe a sense of well-being and satisfaction with their lives. This was described as being related to the presence of trusting relationships with health care providers and therapeutic conversations, as well as antipsychotic medication and family support (Møllerhøj et al., 2019).

Early intervention is thought to be related to better recovery from schizophrenia, especially among those who are experiencing a first psychotic episode (Azrin et al., 2015). One study found that while early intervention, defined as shorter duration of untreated psychotic symptoms, had a positive effect on recovery from schizophrenia, other factors were needed to predict complete recovery. These factors included higher education level, a longer period of employment, and planned medication discontinuation within three together (Chan et al., 2019).

Therapeutic intervention and support play an important role in recovery, which is defined as a personal process of establishing a fulfilling and meaningful life along with a positive sense of identity. Recovery has been found to be promoted by cognitive therapy among individuals suffering from schizophrenia (Vidal & Huguelet, 2019). This demonstrates that psychotherapy can move beyond dealing with specific aspects of schizophrenic disease, to the enhancement of a person's life. A systematic review of cognitive-behavioral and other types of therapy demonstrate they have a positive effect on recovery from schizophrenia (Rakitzi et al., 2020). Later in this book we will describe how there is a good deal of evidence that psychodynamic therapy and psychoanalysis can be effective approaches to helping patients suffering from schizophrenia achieve full recovery as well as increasing the sense of meaning in their lives.

There is still a long way to go in fostering recovery from schizophrenia. Available data indicate that about one in seven people suffering from schizophrenia are able to achieve functional recovery (Silva & Restrepo, 2019). The addition of various types of support, including family support, educational attainment, and psychotherapies could change recovery rates for the better. More research needs to be done on the effectiveness of these modalities on the improvement of recovery.

CHAPTER 10

Prevention of schizophrenia

While prevention of schizophrenia appears to be far-fetched on the surface, many of the latest findings about the disorder provide evidence that preventative approaches may be useful. Environmentally mitigated risk factors related to migration and immigration that are known to increase risk for schizophrenia could be targeted. Exposure to various types of infection could be mitigated or treated. Nutritional risk factors can easily be prevented if adequate and high-quality food supplies are available. Psycho-social stressors, cannabis use, and advanced paternal age, all of which are associated with increased risk for schizophrenia, can be altered to reduce incidence of schizophrenia (A. S. Brown & McGrath, 2011).

There is some evidence that prenatal nutritional deficits increase the risk of schizophrenia. Vitamin D, folic acid, and iron are the three micronutrients that are possibly related to the subsequent development of schizophrenia. Therefore, prenatal supplementation may be protective against the disease (McGrath et al., 2011).

Maternal influenza, toxoplasmosis, and genital/reproductive infections are known to be related to increased risk of schizophrenia in offspring. Prevention of these infections in mothers should be a relatively straight-forward and effective prevention strategy (A. S. Brown & Patterson, 2011).

Possible immunological triggers of schizophrenia, including things that cause gut inflammation and degradation of the gut biome can be avoided, especially among people known to be at higher risk, for example first-degree relatives of patients suffering from schizophrenia (Severance & Yolken, 2020).

New knowledge about schizophrenia has begun to influence how the disorder is treated. In the past, convulsive therapies and psycho-surgery were erroneously thought to be effective treatments for schizophrenia. These invasive and dangerous methods were used often and indiscriminately, causing a great deal of suffering.

Recently, however, greater understanding of the brain, advances in medical technology, and the success of deep brain stimulation (DBS) and psychosurgery for obsessive-compulsive disorder (OCD) have sparked an interest in using these techniques to treat schizo-phrenia. Advanced imaging technology combined with precision surgery now allow for selective targeting of brain structures for neuromodulation via DBS or precise ablation of brain tissue in severe and treatment resistant cases of schizophrenia. These approaches, in an environment of ethical oversight, could lead to important insights about the control of schizophrenic symptoms, while providing treatment options in severe and intractable cases of schizophrenia. Nevertheless, for most people suffering from schizo-phrenia, dopamine modulating antipsychotic medications remain the predominant treatment modality. Both first- and second-generation antipsychotic medications, however, have a number of serious side effects and do not effectively treat the negative and cognitive symptoms associated with schizophrenia.

As a result, novel antipsychotic medications and better medication delivery systems are being developed. Clinical trials have produced mixed results but there is some hope that some of these new approaches will prove as effective or better than previous antipsychotic drugs with fewer side effects. Nevertheless, definitively better antipsychotic pharmacological agents will likely not appear until the pathophysi-ology of schizophrenia is better understood. Another promising area of pharmacological treatment of schizophrenia is anti-inflammatory and immunomodulating agents. A number of these have been studied and there is promise that this approach alone or in conjunction with antipsychotic medication will provide a breakthrough in the treatment and understanding of schizophrenia. While pharmacology continues to be the primary mechanism for treating schizophrenia, psychotherapeutic treatments are showing promise in alleviating some of the debilitating effects of the disease.

Newer psychotherapeutic techniques derived from cognitive-behavioral therapies are showing promise in improving the lives of people suffering from schizophrenia. Innovative formulations of psychodynamic therapies as well as more nuanced understanding of the developmental psychopathology of schizophrenia also show promise in helping to treat the disorder. Many psychotherapies have moved beyond the treatment of symptoms to a focus on recovery. Treatments derived from alternative medicine as well methods of prevention are also being tried or are on the horizon. Even though recovery rates are still low, there is hope that newer therapies as well as the combination of different therapeutic approaches may allow more people suffering from schizophrenia to live happy and fulfilling lives.

Part II

The psychoanalytic metapsychology of schizophrenia

CHAPTER 11

Neuropsychoanalysis and schizophrenia

In order to talk about a psychoanalytic theory and treatment of schizophrenia we need a bridge between the medical and psychological understandings of schizophrenia presented above and current psychoanalytic thinking. An important question to ask is, are the modern biological and psychological understandings of schizophrenia supportive of a psychoanalytic metapsychology of the disease?

Sigmund Freud began his career by proposing, in a work written in 1895, a psychology that would be grounded in a neurophysiological model wherein psychological processes would be able to be quantitatively measured as states in specific material particles (1950a). However, Freud soon gave up this idea and never published his ideas on establishing a psychoanalysis based on neurophysiology. As he later wrote: "But every attempt to go on from there to discover a localization of mental processes, every endeavour to think of ideas as stored up in nerve-cells and of excitations as travelling along nerve-fibres, has miscarried completely" (1915e, p. 174).

Later attempts to combine neurobiology and the perspective of psychoanalytic theory have also fared no better. Robert Cancro, who spoke about biological theories of the human mind, states that such theories are "devoid of psychological content" and "increasingly suffer from reductionism" (1986, p. 106). He was against bastardization of psychoanalytic theories by making them *pseudo-biological*. He said: "Theory can only be useful within a particular realm of discourse, and psychoanalytic theory must function within its assumptions" (p. 106). He hoped that in the future our understanding of the biology of mental activities such as memory and thought would become rich enough to help us shift from the universe of psychology into that of biology with ease. He imagined that when this happened it might be possible to include biological concepts in psychoanalytic theories. This has not yet come about, though progress has been made in creating a robust psychoanalytic metapsychology that allows objective science to meet and inform subjective theoretical and clinical experience (Modell, 1981). Indeed, this continues the tradition begun by Freud of creating maps of the mind that are informed by neuroscience (Kessler & Zellner, 2019).

During the last two decades a significant body of work has emerged to help us toward this goal. As reported above, there are continuing and fascinating findings on brain functions and neurosciences that have, and will have, general relevance for psychoanalysis. For instance, Joshua Roffman and his colleagues (2005) examined the effects of psychotherapy on brain function. Neuroimaging was able to confirm the effects of a number of different types of psychotherapy on brain function across a variety of mental disorders. Other findings have been formulated, studied, or noted by psychoanalysts (Kessler & Zellner, 2019). These studies inform us that new synapses develop in the brain as a result of certain kinds of psychotherapeutic experiences, and they can be verified through brain imaging techniques. They also show us that it is difficult to separate biology from psychology when we examine primitive manifestations of human behavior or behavior associated with severe trauma.

A good example that has relevance for the study of schizophrenia was conducted by Yawei Cheng and colleagues (2010). This study used functional magnetic resonance imaging (fMRI) to see how the brains of people would react when they imagined simulated painful and non-painful stimuli from three perspectives—self, loved ones, and strangers. When subjects took on the perspective of a loved one, they showed increased activity in the anterior cingulate cortex (ACC) and insula. In contrast, taking the perspective of a stranger induced a signal increase in the right-temporo-parietal junction (TPJ) and the superior frontal gyrus. Increased closeness to the loved one induced more deactivation in the TPJ. With imagined strangers, there was negative effective connectivity between the right TPJ and the insula and positive effective connectivity to the superior frontal gyrus. This study clearly shows the connection between the mind and the brain and how they depend on one another. How close one feels to, and how much empathy one has for others, affects a person's brain.

Brian Johnson and Daniela Flores Mosri (2016) relate these findings to psychotherapy:

> Apart from it showing correlates between the quality of relationships and neuroanatomical structures, which is another piece of evidence of how the mind and brain depend upon each other and are influenced by experience, it also alerts the psychoanalyst that the state of the countertransference may influence the accuracy of empathy. How close one feels to one's patient influences the brain of the psychoanalyst. (p. 2)

It is easy to imagine the reverse situation as well. The quality of transference to the analyst will be affected by how close the patient feels to the therapist as well. The authors go on to discuss the neurobiology of the pain system and how patients taking opioids, or those who have low opioid tone due to early attachment issues will have a flattened emotional response. They comment that:

> A neurobiologically informed psychodynamic psychotherapist might be able to better apply transference-based techniques with patients who show compromised object relations such as borderline states by taking into account a probable chronic low opioid tone which is a product of early childhood attachment patterns. (p. 3)

Since opioids interact with the dopaminergic system in the brain this type of insight may have clinical relevance for patients suffering from schizophrenia and may provide insight on how to better conduct effective psychotherapy with them. This may be especially relevant for

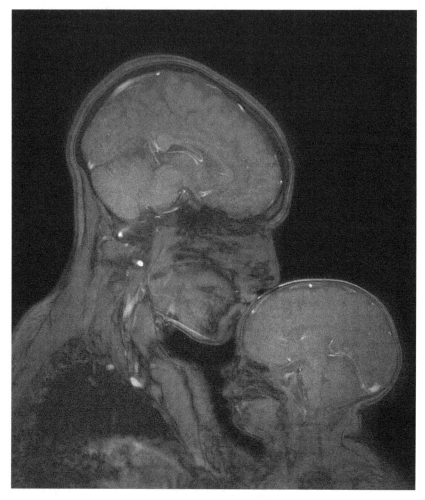

Figure 1 MRI image of mother and child (Rebecca Saxe and Atsushi Takahashi/Department of Brain and Cognitive Sciences, MIT/ Athinoula A. Martinos Imaging Center at the McGovern Institute for Brain Research, MIT).

the development of psychotherapy techniques for working with patients suffering from schizophrenia who are chronically medicated with neuroleptic drugs.

In an article for *Smithsonian Magazine*, Massachusetts Institute of Technology neuroscientist Rebecca Saxe published an MRI image of her holding her infant son (Saxe, 2015). In the image, we can clearly see a mother bonding with her child while we observe the brains of each. This picture is a wonderful metaphor of psychoanalytic metapsychology— that our mental development begins with our earliest relationships and that this interaction is intimately related to the structural growth of our brains. Indeed, Saxe's research involves using MRI imagery to see how brain activity changes with people's thoughts. This type of research is now increasingly being used in conjunction with psychoanalytic theory. Neurobiology and brain structure are being related to thoughts, which leads to insights about the nature of mind, which is in turn influenced by relationships with external people and environments. Stefano Marini and his colleagues (2016) review a number of excellent examples of how this type of fMRI work has been used in psychoanalysis.

These types of imaging studies support research that looks at how the external world impacts brain development and the pathogenesis of schizophrenia. For instance, Pekka Tienari and his colleagues' findings from their research project in Oulu, Finland on twins and adopted children (Wahlberg et al., 1997). These investigators concluded that attempting to assess the respective importance of genetic (biological) vulnerability and family environment is futile. Influences come from either direction. Adopted children at high risk are more likely to develop schizophrenia if the family is clearly dysfunctional. Other research on early baby-mother interactions, also in Finland, shows that in such interactions biology and psychology become intertwined (Lehtonen, 2003; Lehtonen et al., 2002; Purhonen et al., 2001).

Studies like these demonstrate that brain structures, as well as attachment and memory, can be affected by the external environment, which not only includes traumas but also psychotherapeutic treatment processes. This serves as the backdrop for the development of psychoanalytic theories of schizophrenia.

CHAPTER 12

Early psychoanalytic approaches to understanding schizophrenia

This chapter reviews some key psychoanalytic concepts concerning schizophrenia, a mental condition that is difficult to place under one clear diagnostic category. While starting with Sigmund Freud, the focus here is on psychoanalysts in the United States and their psychoanalytic considerations on this subject.

Nathaniel London (1973a, 1973b) classified Freud's contributions on schizophrenia in adults under two incompatible models, the "specific theory" and the "unitary theory." Freud (1911c, 1914d, 1915e) used ideas outside of his theory of neuroses in order to specifically understand the psychodynamics of schizophrenia and this became known as the specific theory. Later, Freud explained both the neurotic and schizophrenic categories of pathology utilizing one and the same theory (1924b, 1924e), which became known as the unitary theory.

Freud's *specific theory* focuses on the withdrawal of libido from the object and the transformation of psychic energy from the object to the "ego." Using current terminology, we can say that libido is withdrawn from the object representation, which is a collection of many images pertaining to the object and transformed to self-representation. This results in megalomania and hypochondriasis. Freud postulated that after the withdrawal, the person reestablishes contact with the outside world in a restitutional effort, which itself is pathological and is characterized by delusions and hallucinations. The specific theory is also known as the *libidinal decathexis–recathexis* process. Decathexis is experienced as a "*world destruction fantasy*" and recathexis is experienced as a "*world construction fantasy*" (Fenichel, 1945). Most patients exhibit symptoms associated with *both* decathexis and recathexis.

Freud's specific theory does not inform us as to how and why each transformation (decathexis and recathexis) occurs. Among its failures to explain schizophrenic conditions, the theory contains two major omissions: First, it does not indicate how the nature of the object itself (or its representation) plays a role in the evolution of schizophrenia. Second, there is no reference to the presence of aggression as an essential aspect of psychological processes, or an understanding of how both self- and object representations become invested with aggression.

Freud's *unitary theory* of schizophrenia came a year after he published *The Ego and the Id* (1923b) and established the structural theory of psychoanalysis. Nathaniel London's description of Freud's unitary theory refers to the intrapsychically motivated behavior arising from *drives* and defenses against drive expressions witnessed in individuals with *both* neuroses and psychoses (London, 1973a, 1973b). However, it was Heinz Hartmann's (1939) revision of Freud's structural theory that effectively added new ideas about Freud's second reformulation of his ideas about schizophrenia.

Hartmann assigned to the ego its own primary (libidinal as well as aggressive) psychic energy and made it a structure of the mind that has its own autonomous functions. This so-called "ego psychology" is primarily based on Hartmann's revised structural theory. Hartmann emphasized that the symptoms associated with schizophrenia could be understood as a *selective* regression or progression of some ego functions (1954). This explained the wide range and lack of uniformity of symptoms among people suffering from schizophrenia (Pao, 1979).

In the United States, during the days when "ego psychology" was dominant, the application of the structural theory to our understanding of schizophrenia received support from many psychoanalytic theoreticians. Jacob Arlow and Charles Brenner (1964) spoke of selective regression and modifications in certain ego and superego functions. They believed that drive regression also exists to a greater extent in schizophrenia than in neurotic pathology.

Nevertheless, some analysts continued to apply the structural theory when understanding and treating people with neurotic personality organization, while returning to Freud's specific theory concepts of decathexis–recathexis in understanding and treating people who develop schizophrenia as teens or young adults. A good example of this can be found in Otto Fenichel's (1945) classic book, *The Psychoanalytic Theory of Neurosis*. He used the terminology of structural theory to describe the neurotic personality but adhered to the specific theory with its libidinal decathexis–recathexis model in describing schizo- phrenia. One of the reasons many analysts held on to the specific theory for so long was because it is internally consistent, explaining the meaning of schizophrenic symptoms well. As stated above, the specific theory fails in that it ignores certain key considerations, such as the role aggression plays in the evolution and maintenance of primitive mental states.

Applying the unitary theory with its structural model, including the version that developed after Heinz Hartmann's work (1939, 1954), to conflicts experienced by adults with schizophrenia also proved to be problematic. One simple reason is that adults suffering from schizo- phrenia do not have a fully differentiated tripartite (id, ego, superego) structural apparatus; and certainly, their superegos are not fully formed, and their egos have deficiencies. The "superego," which is fully developed after the resolution of the Oedipus complex, does not fit into a metapsychology explaining the internal world of a teenager or a young adult suffering from schizophrenia. One way of under- standing the superego lack of fit with the etiology of schizophrenia was to add adjectives when describing superegos of individuals suffering from schizophrenia using terms such as "precursors of the superego" or "archaic superego." Furthermore, the structural theory does not easily explain or cannot explain clinical observations pertaining to ego deficiencies, neither can it explain identity confusion and diffusion, object hunger, or the clashing of terrifying and/or idealized and simul- taneously fragmented self- and object images. In addition, this theory could not clearly illuminate developmental issues observed during clinical practice.

Nevertheless, the application of ego psychology to the understanding of the etiology of schizophrenia continued. However, some psychoanalysts in the United States, such as Harry Stack Sullivan (1962) and Frieda Fromm-Reichmann (1939, 1959), who were involved in the treatment of persons suffering from schizophrenia in long-term inpatient facilities, began to notice that patients suffering from schizophrenia were capable of developing intense transference manifestations. This ran counter to Freud's belief that such patients were incapable of this kind of transference reaction.

Sullivan and his followers focused on early interpersonal difficulties in child–parent relationships among those who would develop adult schizophrenia, and on the anxiety conveyed to them by their mothers or other mothering persons during their early developmental years. Fromm-Reichmann, rather unfortunately, referred to *schizophrenogenic* mothers. Later it became clear that there is no specific personality type among the mothers of people suffering from schizophrenia. Nevertheless, Fromm-Reichmann brought to our attention the existence of various poisonous mother–child interactions that are found among some individuals suffering from schizophrenia, while Theodore Lidz and Stephen Fleck (1960) focused on the whole family's role in the etiology of schizophrenia in one of its members.

In 1953, Anna Freud, with then well-known psychoanalysts Edith Jacobson, Edith Weigert, and Leo Stone, discussed the "widening scope of psychoanalysis." During this discussion, she asked:

> How do analysts decide if they are given the choice between returning to health half a dozen young people with good prospects in life but disturbed in their enjoyment and efficiency by comparatively mild neuroses, or to devote the same time, trouble and effort to one single borderline case, who may or may not be saved from spending the rest of his life in an institution? (A. Freud, 1954, pp. 610–611)

Anna Freud's bias was toward treating *only* neurotic patients instead of struggling with new technical problems.

But a group of analysts and others in the United States such as Andreas Angyal (1950), Bryce Boyer (1961, 1971, 1983), Donald Burnham (Burnham et al., 1969), Peter Giovacchini (1969, 1972), James Grotstein (1986), Ping-Nie Pao (1979), Clarence Schulz (1983), Harold Searles (1959, 1961, 1979, 1986), Vamık Volkan (1976, 1986, 1990, 1994, 1995, 2015a) and Otto Will (1964), slowly made the psychoanalytic and psychoanalytically oriented treatment of persons with schizophrenia, whether their conditions started during the developmental years, teenage, or young adulthood years, an acceptable practice within American psychoanalytic circles. This occurred in spite of resistance from the dominant ego psychology position in psychoanalysis that insisted that severely regressed persons were unsuitable for psychoanalysis. Recently, other psychoanalytic clinicians have shown that evidence-based psychoanalytic treatment modalities are effective in treating people suffering from schizophrenia (Downing & Mills, 2018; Garfield & Mackler, 2013; Gibbs, 2007).

Harold Searles, who was especially influenced by Margaret Mahler's (1952) work with autistic or symbiotic infantile psychosis, thought that in adult schizophrenia an ego regression occurs to a level that "has its prototype in the experience of the young infant for whom inner and outer worlds have not yet become clearly distinguishable as such" (Searles, 1961, p. 525). This new group of psychoanalysts' therapeutic involvement with adults with schizophrenia and other severely regressed individuals taught that a psychoanalytic approach helps to modify the internal structures of people suffering from schizophrenia. Experience in treating individuals suffering from schizophrenia provided information about the primitive functions of the mind and its metapsychological considerations. This led to an extension of the theoretical and treatment approaches to schizophrenia championed by psychoanalysts and psychoanalytically oriented therapists in other countries, such as Melanie Klein in England and Yrjö Alanen in Finland and their followers.

Boyer, Giovacchini, Searles and others' works with adults with schizophrenia also brought necessary attention to countertransference issues and to the so-called "two-person psychology" that is the contemporary buzzword in today's culture of pluralism in American psychoanalysis—as if there had ever been a "one-person psychology" in psychoanalytic practice. Focus on object relations increased. Interestingly, most of the clinicians and theoreticians in the United States mentioned above adhered to the key principles of ego psychology, while also helping to expand the application of object relations theories.

CHAPTER 13

A review of object relations and severe psychopathology

Following Edith Jacobson's (1964) work, Otto Kernberg (1966, 1976, 1984) offered a version of object relations theory that increased the psychoanalytic tools for examining the inner worlds of adults with various severe psychopathologies. Kernberg himself perceived adults with schizophrenia or psychotic personality organization as being untreatable by psychoanalysis and/or psycho-analytic psychotherapy. He focused primarily on the psychoanalytic treatment of persons with borderline and/or narcissistic personality organizations. Kernberg saw drives as attached to different images or representations of self and objects with their associated peak affective expressions. His theory brought a focus on the differentiation and integration functions of the ego.

First let us examine *differentiation*. It refers to the differentiation of self-images from object images and is the basis of the separation between self and other. The second ego function involves the *integration* of the differentiated "good" (libidinally invested) self-images with the differentiated "bad" (aggressively invested) self-images, as well as the integration of differentiated "good" object images with differentiated "bad" object images. This is the basis of ambivalence—the ability to experience others and one's self as both good and bad. Individuals accomplishing both functions are those who have reached a "high-level" (neurotic) personality organization. If adults are considered as having a narcissistic or borderline personality organization, it can be said that they have achieved the ability to perform the first ego function albeit poorly at times, while having failed, to one extent or another, to acquire the second one. For people who have a schizo-phrenic condition, none of the two ego functions are available to them at a functional level.

Otto Kernberg's theory refers to object relations conflicts, and this drastically differentiates his theory from self psychology developed by Heinz Kohut (1971) around the same time. Kohut's theory focuses on the self, but not on conflicts. Individuals with neuroses are aware, or can be made aware during psychoanalysis, that internal conflicts belong to them; all the opposing tendencies are internally motivated. Individuals who are caught up in object relations conflict can feel tension between the split or fragmented self-images, but more often they experience tension between their own desires and the prohibitions, injunctions, and values assigned to their internalized (or externalized) images of other people that sometimes are fused with unintegrated self-images (Dorpat, 1976). People with object relations conflicts therefore do not own, or fully own, their internal conflicts. They feel tensions between themselves and "others" who represent their internalized or externalized selves and object images. Some of these "others" are representations of patients' externalized "superego forerunners" or the "archaic superego."

Stanley Greenspan and Beryl Benderly (1997) challenged object relations theory as systematized by Kernberg, stating that it informed us little about the concept of "deficiency" of ego functions during early development and its causes. Greenspan wrote about both early deficiencies and conflicts in the formation of psychopathology and, not unlike other researchers who study the evolution of an infant's mind, postulated that infants are pre-wired. These researchers believe that this pre-wiring can organize experiences with the mother in the early weeks or months of life, setting the stage for higher levels of personality organization to develop later. The term "mother" should also include those who are involved in a dyadic mothering relationship with the child.

Not all infants are alike; some may be hyper-arousable while others are hypo-arousable. Some may have difficulty integrating different sensory pathways, such as vision and hearing. This underlines the importance of a "fit" between the infant and the mother (Emde, 1988a, 1988b; Lehtonen et al., 2002). Many things can undermine this fit, including a large number of the risk factors for schizophrenia outlined above.

Psychoanalytic structural theory is still the best instrument for understanding the psychopathology of patients with fully differentiated id, ego, and superego functions (V. Volkan, 1981). Nevertheless, when treating persons whose dominant psychopathology reflects the reactivation of internalized object relation conflicts, structural theory alone is no longer adequate. The use of object relations theory is more effective in better understanding patients' psychological processes until they arrive at the neurotic level during their treatment. It is generally agreed that the primacy of repression and related defense mechanisms operating in individuals with neurotic personality organization becomes replaced by the primacy of splitting and related defense mechanisms such as externalization and internalization (more about these terms follows below) of such images that are seen in persons with borderline or narcissistic personality organization.

We should note that the term splitting used here does not refer to splitting an ego mechanism such as when a woman in acute grief who knows that her husband had just died but who also "hears" her husband is parking his car in front of the family house. Here splitting refers to separating self and object images saturated with libido from self and object images saturated with aggression. The focus on splitting of self and object images and related defense mechanisms helped psychoanalysts come up with modified psychoanalytic techniques in the treatment of individuals with borderline or narcissistic personality organization (Kernberg, 1975, 1984; V. Volkan, 1987, 2010).

But this new knowledge about primitive-level object relations was not utilized as a guideline or as a new motivation for more psychoanalysts to try to treat adults with schizophrenia. The object relations dynamics of people suffering from schizophrenia involve defensive internalization–externalization, fusion-disconnecting, and uniting-fragmentation cycles of self- and object images that overshadow defensive splitting. In our early writings, instead of using the expression "internalization–externalization cycle," we called these activities an "introjection-projection cycle." In this book, in order to separate object relations of individuals suffering from schizophrenia from typical introjections and projections of thoughts, attitudes, tasks, affects as well as self and object images utilized by individuals with higher-level personality organizations, we chose to stay with the term "internalization–externalization cycle." The continuing fear among analysts was that individuals suffering from schizophrenia would develop unmanageable, dangerous, and unworkable psychotic transferences. In short, the availability of object relations theory in the 1960s and 1970s and the decades that followed did not bring about an increase in the number of psychoanalysts or other types of therapists working with adults suffering from schizophrenia.

In any case, beginning in the 1970s, several other factors were responsible for relegating psychoanalytic treatment of adults with schizophrenia to something of the past. These factors included a shift to biological focus in psychiatry and psychology, changes in the reimbursement systems for psychological treatment, legal worries concerning malpractice, and the closure of most of the well-known psychoanalytically oriented hospitals and inpatient facilities (with some exceptions such as the Austen Riggs Center, which is still open).

On the seemingly bright side, there was a revival of interest in psychoanalysis coinciding with the opening of psychoanalytic training to non-MD practitioners. This revitalized psychoanalysis and created an atmosphere of pluralism where many new ideas and theories began to flourish in the field. However, the downside to these positive changes in psychoanalysis was that various competing and even incompatible ideas and technical considerations began to overshadow some of the fundamental tenets of psychoanalysis. Some object relations theorists and practitioners abandoned the necessity of drives as the motivating force for early psychodynamics, substituting instead an innate need for relationship. This resulted in so-called "soft" object relations schools where attention to the unconscious factors in pathology is unfortunately minimized. The result of these changes is that, for all practical purposes, psychoanalysts, as well as other kinds of psychotherapists, in the United States "stopped" treating people with schizophrenia using a psychodynamic approach.

The proverbial baby was thrown out with the bathwater. This is unfortunate especially given that neurobiology, pharmacology, and newer cognitive forms of psychotherapy have been unsuccessful in doing more than alleviating the symptoms of schizophrenia. A theory of the etiology of schizophrenia, explicated using psychoanalytic metapsychology based on early object relations dynamics, is able to provide treatment techniques for some people suffering from schizophrenia and, hopefully, inspire the development of new treatments for others who suffer from this debilitating syndrome.

CHAPTER 14

Schizophrenic etiology and organismal panic

As a background to these views of the etiology of schizophrenia, it is possible to start with Ping-Nie Pao's (1979) understanding of how adult schizophrenia begins. Pao agreed with the ego psychologists that prone teenagers or young adults suffering from schizophrenia deal with the same kinds of conflicts as people with neuroses do. When some life events awaken repressed conflicts in schizophrenia-prone individuals, they lead to organismic panic instead of ordinary signal anxiety. Pao's term "organismic panic" was based on Margaret Mahler's "organismic distress," (Mahler & Furer, 1968) describing that physiological state of high tension experienced by an infant for whom the mothering person can provide relief.

Allan Schore (2015) describes something similar along with its neurological correlates in the psychotic breaks of people suffering from borderline personality disorder or schizophrenic relapse. The distress is associated with orbitofrontal cortex shifting from hyper to hypo activity and a loss of regulation through a subcortical ergotropic arousal followed by trophotropic arousal. These states are associated with the emotions of anxiety and humiliation as well as a contraction and disappearance of nearby visual space. As Schore reports: "Indeed, the mental states that occur at the peak of ergotropic and trophotropic arousal have been described as timeless and spaceless. These findings suggest that the state transition of the black hole phenomenon may represent a terrifying portal through which the borderline descends into psychotic states" (p. 422).

Ping-Nie Pao noted that the organismic panic is of short duration and it includes a shock where the ego's integrative function becomes paralyzed. Allan Schore (2015) also describes this paralysis along with the loss of capacity for speech. Soon after, the integrative function is restored, but not at a mature level, and the organismic panic ends. The person's "recovery" becomes associated with a regression in perceptual-cognitive-motor processes, along with the reactivation of more primitive defense mechanisms. The patient perceives the experience of self in this regressed state as an internal personality change. Then, the schizophrenic condition is crystallized around the changed personality (Sandler & Joffe, 1969).

Consistent with what Pao observed, the conflicts experienced by schizophrenia-prone adults in their teen years or early adulthood are not identical to the conflicts that exist in people of the same age group with neuroses (V. Volkan, 1995). Unlike people suffering from neurosis, schizophrenia-prone individuals' conflicts are primarily object relations conflicts. Although schizophrenia-prone people sometimes seem preoccupied with structural conflicts, exhibit oedipal issues and castration anxiety like individuals with neuroses, a closer examination of their internal worlds reveals that they are defensively "reaching up" (Boyer, 1983) to higher-level concerns in order to escape the tensions created by their object relations conflicts. While Pao rightly referred to a personality change following the organismic panic, he did not provide detailed information on the typical features of such a changed personality.

Many teenagers or young adults who develop schizophrenia are capable of describing how they perceive the changes in their internal worlds as they enter into schizophrenia. James Glass's (1985) study of the psychological breakdown of the inner world of adults entering schizophrenia and experiencing an organismic panic is a classic. He describes, for example, patients feeling that a star is exploding into millions of pieces within them. His observations correspond to the classical observations on the so-called "world destruction fantasies" (Fenichel, 1945) seen at

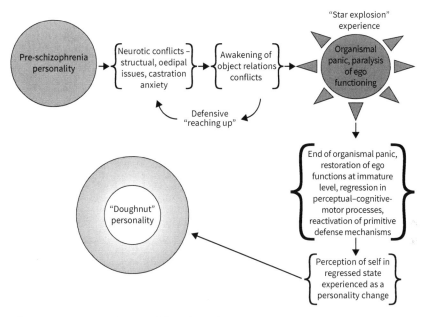

Figure 2 Descent into schizophrenia.

the onset of adult schizophrenia. James Grotstein (1990a, 1990b, 1991) similarly reports on the "black hole" experience of those descending into psychosis.

"Doughnut personality"

In order to describe these ideas on the etiology of schizophrenia, it is instructive to focus on patients' descriptions of their personality changes soon after this so-called "star-explosion" event, and the loss of their existing personality. These patients, at least for a short time, describe a new personality, which can be described as a "doughnut personality." This doughnut analogy refers to patients' experience of an exaggeratedly fearsome or exaggeratedly idealized outer layer, which is the "dough" of the doughnut, and a middle part that is either perceived as empty or filled with unpalatable "bad" jelly. These patients suffering from schizophrenia experience the outer layer as a "monster" or the opposite, an "angel" (or some similar term) according to the degree to which this component is saturated with the derivatives of aggression or libido.

Sometimes the "monster" alternates with the "angel." They describe the second component "in the middle" as a place filled with "bad" affects, reflecting terms used long ago by some clinicians or researchers, such as "anaclitic depression" (Spitz, 1965). Patients may call this second component their "bad seed." When they totally deny unnamable affects and/or derivatives of aggression, they may say that their middle core is an area of "emptiness."

The intensity of the organismic panic changes from case to case. Furthermore, because of the extensive use of antipsychotic drugs at the present time there are only rare opportunities to observe teenagers or young adults going into schizophrenia and listening to detailed descriptions of their personality change. What can be gleaned from them is clouded by medications that create numbness or physical symptoms such as tardive dyskinesia that require even further medication.

Patients descending into schizophrenia often described two components of the "doughnut personality." After a while, the outer component of the dough changes; a sense of extra omnipotence (megalomania) infiltrates the dough. For example, patients now declare that they are Jesus or another prophet, the greatest musician, or the best terrorist. This corresponds to classical observations on the development of "world construction fantasies." But here what is being described is a new construction in these patients' perceived sense of their internal world. When their omnipotence settles, references to the "bad seed" or "emptiness" seem to lessen a great deal or disappear altogether.

The experience of a mental hospital patient suffering from schizo-phrenia named Juan exemplifies this doughnut dynamic. Juan was an illiterate farmworker of Peruvian descent. He would stand outside in the hospital yard staring at the sky. When asked what he was looking at, he described a magnificent crystal Incan city arranged in a circle, with beautiful buildings and inhabited by celestial gods and beings. However, in the center of this was a terrifying void. A long string of beads extended from this void down from the sky to Juan, trying to pull him inside while he resisted. Juan, paralyzed by (organismal) panic, reported that he had to keep looking at the crystal city in order not to be pulled into the dangerous emptiness. A few weeks later, Juan was no longer concerned about the void and instead reported that he was Jesus and that he lived in the crystal city.

Another example was a schizophrenic sufferer named Sam. He had been affected by the sight of a woman in a passionate embrace with another man—a woman for whom he had a strong romantic attachment without any encouragement from her. In reality Sam had object relations conflicts, and the woman he loved from a distance represented both his "good" and "bad" mother. Soon thereafter Sam had a dream in which his home city was bombed and later, while awake and driving his car, he "saw" a mushroom cloud rise up ahead of him. His horror at the sight led him to drive into a ditch, screaming with terror (organismic panic). Taken to a hospital, he looked like a terrified animal. He explained what had happened, saying that although he knew that the atomic bomb had exploded over the city, he felt it explode within his body as well. Sam also referred to himself as a monster. After a month in the hospital, he was discharged into the care of his family. However, he was returned to the hospital two months later, appearing much calmer, but called himself "Saint Sam" and claiming a new, omnipotent, and religious identity.

Jim, a philosophy graduate student at a state university, began to suffer overwhelming terror after a female professor critiqued a paper he had written. His professor, whom he both idolized and feared, represented both a good and bad mother. Jim checked himself into a private hospital but refused medication. His first days on the ward consisted of Jim having philosophical arguments with various voices or people he hallucinated. Jim reported that these interminable arguments seemed to help defend against feelings of overwhelming terror and the feeling that he would explode. The arguments became more and more heated and hostile, with Jim referring to himself as a fiend or a freak. After a few weeks, however, the tenor of the arguments began to change. Jim's arguments became more of a coherent discussion of how great a philosopher he was and how he was the only one who understood and could find solutions to unsolvable philosophical problems. At this time Jim became much calmer and easier for staff to deal with. He eventually accepted medication and was discharged and returned to his studies at the university.

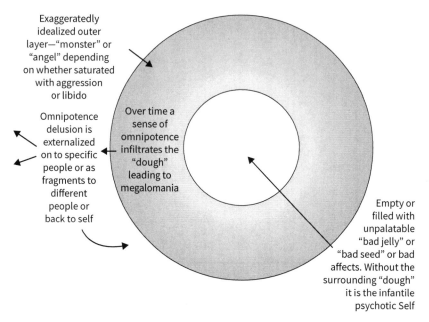

Exaggeratedly idealized outer layer—"monster" or "angel" depending on whether saturated with aggression or libido

Omnipotence delusion is externalized on to specific people or as fragments to different people or back to self

Over time a sense of omnipotence infiltrates the "dough" leading to megalomania

Empty or filled with unpalatable "bad jelly" or "bad seed" or bad affects. Without the surrounding "dough" it is the infantile psychotic Self

Figure 3 "Doughnut personality" or adult psychotic self.

Patients like these later continue exhibiting omnipotence, or their sense of omnipotence may become hidden through the utilization of externalizations of megalomania on single or multiple objects. For example, after a time of being a "doughnut" the patient experiences himself or herself as Jesus Christ or Mother Theresa and then someone out there becomes Christ or Mother Theresa in the patient's delusion, and the patient evolves as a follower. Or Christ or Mother Theresa is divided into various segments and these segments are externalized onto others or sometimes kept within.

Clinical observations like these led to the theoretical concept of "the adult psychotic self" and "the infantile psychotic self." Briefly, the total doughnut is the adult psychotic self (V. Volkan, 1995; V. Volkan & Akhtar, 1997). It exists in every adult person with schizophrenia and its existence is necessary for a psychoanalytic metapsychological diagnosis of adult schizophrenia. If the outer layer's omnipotence can be maintained, the patient does not perceive the "bad" jelly or emptiness. The adult psychotic self is an indication that the patient has gone through—after experiencing an organismic panic and after the explosion of the internal world—a drastic personality change. The infantile psychotic self is the jelly filled with unnamable "bad" affect *without* dough around it. It will be useful to examine the concept of the infantile psychotic self first, before examining the establishment of an adult psychotic self and other related conditions.

CHAPTER 15

The infantile psychotic self

It is puzzling why some teenagers or young adults are prone to having organismic panic instead of signal anxiety and then, following an organismic panic, going through a personality change. Such phenomena cannot be explained by focusing on these individuals' ego, superego, or drive regressions alone. In order to explain organismic panic and personality change leading to schizophrenia it is possible to postulate the existence of an "infantile psychotic self," or what can be called a "seed of madness" in schizophrenia-prone adults (V. Volkan & Akhtar, 1997). It is possible to observe such "seeds" at a close range when they appear in the transference psychosis of adult individuals suffering from schizophrenia, as well as some of psychosis-prone individuals suffering from borderline personality disorder (V. Volkan, 1964, 1976, 1986, 1990, 1994, 1995; V. Volkan & Akhtar, 1979, 1997).

The minds of babies and children evolve and are formed through stimulation of existing psychobiological and species-specific (Tähkä, 1993) potentials during interactions with their environment. Psychologically speaking, this environment is a restricted one, consisting of the mother or others who provide mothering functions. It is possible to imagine the early child–mother interaction as represented by a test tube in which many ingredients, what Sigmund Freud (1914d) called "disposition and experience" (p. 18), are mixed. When this mixture comes out from this test tube it represents the child's core infantile self. This core self can be healthy due to the libidinalization of the mixture, or can become "psychotic" due to the saturation of the mixture with aggression. Both growth-stimulating and growth-inhibiting ingredients come from the child as well as from the mother, whether they are biological, epigenetic, genetic, and structural or psychological. These ingredients influence the nature of the mixture and the associated mind-building process. In some cases, non-psychological flawed ingredients are dominant. For example, a child may be born with a physiological or genetic condition that would interfere with the development of an ego function that tames aggression.

As discussed above, we now know more about the influences of genetics and, perhaps more importantly, epigenetics on early development. We are now seeing the creation of biomolecular models of how both genes and genetic expression can be related to schizophrenia. In particular, a number of studies have demonstrated how the three epigenetic mechanisms that regulate gene expression (DNA methylation, histone modifications, and micro RNAs) can go awry in people suffering from schizophrenia. Some if not many of the elements of epigenetic dysregulation of gene expression in schizophrenia are due in part to environmental insults (flawed ingredients) that are experienced in the pre- and postnatal periods by the mother or the child.

Many of the ingredients related to the development of schizophrenia in humans, such as exposure to infectious disease, neurobiological pathologies, autoimmune dysfunction, etc., may have some relationship to epigenetics, which we have discussed in detail above. Psychoanalysis and neuroscience share an emphasis on the effects of the early developmental period as the root of severe pathology such as schizophrenia. As Tamara Fischmann (2016) puts it, "These epigenetic factors control genomic functions by turning genes on or off, depending on, for instance, early childhood experiences of maltreatment" (p. 102). Both fields see the possibility for inducing normative epigenetic changes as a potential treatment strategy (Gibbs, 2007; Leuzinger-Bohleber, 2016). Neuroscientists have mostly suggested bringing about normative gene expression through epigenetically targeted pharmacology. Psychoanalysis and psychoanalytic therapy may be able to induce similar epigenetic changes either alone or in concert with newer pharmacological treatments (Gorman, 2016). A study by Huango Colangeli (2020) suggests that since psychoanalysis has proved successful in treating intergenerational trauma, and that changes in DNA expression can be transmitted between generations, it is possible that psychoanalytic treatment could positively affect DNA expression.

It is a misconception to believe that psychoanalysts and psychoanalytic therapists discount these factors and ascribe the genesis of schizophrenia solely as the result of psychological factors. It is important to acknowledge that the causes of schizophrenia discussed in the sections above are important and that schizophrenia can have its origins in these biological, epigenetic, genetic, and structural factors. It is crucial for psychoanalytic clinicians and theorists to have some understanding of the factors related to the development of schizophrenia, which is why we have presented them above. However, as we have seen, the distinction between these factors is a gray area and there are many overlapping complex interactions. Specifically, some biological and epigenetic factors can be directly influenced by psychological factors and vice versa. And these biological and epigenetic factors have an intimate relationship with genetic and structural factors. Therefore, it is also a misconception to discount the effect of psychoanalysis and psychoanalytic therapy on the non-psychological factors.

In the future, it is likely that research will elucidate more closely the causal relationship between the genetic, epigenetic, psychological, and structural factors involved in the genesis of schizophrenia. What is being postulated here is that the biological, epigenetic, genetic, and structural factors then must be necessarily associated with the psychological factors that are involved in the development of the schizophrenic personality. Unfortunately, the psychological factors related to the genesis of schizophrenia have been minimized in the fields of psychiatry and psychology, yet they are extremely important in order to understand and treat schizophrenia as well as give an empathetic sense of the phenomenology of those who suffer from such a devastating diagnosis. Therefore, this work will focus on the psychological factors, a subset of the so-called flawed ingredients, observed by the authors and others.

CHAPTER 16

Flawed ingredients

Child disappearance fantasy

The first such psychologically flawed ingredient refers to a mother's unconscious fantasy that her child should disappear or die (see also Apprey, 1997). The mother's unconscious fantasy is passed on to the patient suffering from schizophrenia who experiences it in the following way: "My mother did not wish me to be born. I should get rid of my self-image (or representation) or mind in order to please my mother. This will give me hope to have a better mother who will love me. On the other hand, I will not exist; I will have a psychological death."

Patients suffering from schizophrenia do not have such sentences in their minds, of course; the experience takes place at a preverbal level. However, through the observation of relationships of patients suffering from schizophrenia with the external world and their transference psychosis, it is possible to infer that some patients suffering from schizophrenia have such experiences. Later, such patients will be able to verbalize these thought processes after achieving a higher-level personality organization during their treatment. But even the patients' initial histories and/or behavior patterns can be informative about the existence of a mother's death wish for her child and the child's corresponding unconscious fantasy. For example, there may be a family history in which the mother did not know that she was pregnant until the seventh month of her pregnancy. Or there may be a family story in which the patient was conceived a week prior to the mother's planned surgery to have her tubes tied. The patient may have a history of multiple suicide attempts. Or the patient may have tried to change his or her name or carve a new name on her body. The patient may have repeating dreams of disappearing or delusions of having other parents or of being brought to earth from outer space.

Borderline or psychotic mothering

If the mother suffers from psychosis or severe borderline personality organization, she may not be able to provide the necessary initial libidinalization of the baby's infantile core self. In other words, the baby will not build up enough pleasurable experiences with the mother to facilitate the development of a healthy self-representation. Some mothers do not have a reasonable "fit" between their own activities and temperament and those of their child (Brazelton & Greenspan, 2000; Greenspan & Benderly, 1997).

To paraphrase Donald Winnicott (1953) the mothering is not "good enough" and the experience of persecutory internal object representations is enhanced. Joyce McDougall (1986) and Marita Torsti (1998), in a sense reflecting Frieda Fromm-Reichmann's (1959) old schizophrenogenic mother image, spoke of addictive and oral mothers respectively in referring to women who cling to their children and in turn "murder" the child's developing mind. Other mothers present mental functions to the child that create "inassimilable contradictions" (Burnham et al., 1969, p. 55) leading to the building up of aggressive "bad" affects in the child's infantile core self.

Handicap effects

Sometimes handicaps such as blindness in the baby or mother become negative ingredients in the metaphorical "test tube" that we described earlier. Obviously, such handicaps alone in a mother or an infant do not lead to schizophrenia in the child during childhood or adulthood. But at times such physical disabilities may prevent the development of certain ego functions in the child, and this may become a negative element within the "test tube." It is possible to speculate more subtle physical malfunctions due to infection, or autoimmunity and inflammation may affect the development of the ego in addition to more overt physical disabilities. How the mother handles the child's physical problems can play a crucial role in either supporting normal psychological development or promoting psychopathology.

For example, a patient, Ricky, was born with a deformed hand and fingers. This was a blow to his mother's narcissism. As she was not able to libidinalize her baby's infantile core self, she denied her child's handicap. From his early childhood, she gave Ricky a golden ring every year for his birthday, rings that would not fit his deformed fingers. The mother, through this and other similar behavior patterns, could not help Ricky establish a realistic body image and learn about reality testing. We will talk more about Ricky's case in Chapter 20.

Having a handicapped sibling can be another negative factor. The grieving mother may neglect or overprotect the physically normal child (Colonna & Newman, 1983; V. Volkan & Ast, 1997), creating a negative element in the child's mind-building. Raising a surviving twin, or a surviving child after the death of previous children, may have a strong pathogenic impact on a mother's relationship with her child (K. Volkan, 1994).

Transitional objects

A mother's interference with the normal development of the child's transitional objects or phenomena is another negative ingredient. For example, the mother becomes envious of the baby's preoccupation with a teddy bear and hides the toy or discards it without giving the baby an opportunity to develop a transitional phenomenon or create another transitional object. The mother may repeat her behavior pattern. The normal evolution of the transitional object and phenomenon and the child's normal play with them are necessary for the child's getting to know the surrounding environment (Winnicott, 1953). Such play with transitional objects ushers in reality testing (Greenacre, 1970).

Adult individuals with schizophrenia, especially those with mothers who intruded in their maintaining and playing with transitional objects or phenomena, will, during psychoanalytic treatment, use the analyst as a transitional object in a certain period of their transference relationship. They will also actually play with newly created transitional objects or phenomena in the external world, sometimes giving up their previous reactivated pathological transitional objects and phenomena. For example, Maria, a woman in her late twenties, during a certain phase of her treatment with Vamık Volkan, became preoccupied with learning Turkish tunes and playing them on the piano (she knew that her analyst is of Turkish origin) and gave up a dirty handkerchief (a pathologically recreated transitional object) she had been carrying with her everywhere since her post-pubertal years.

For people suffering from schizophrenia, who have achieved the differentiation function of the ego but lack rudimentary integration of good and bad object representations, the internalization–externalization cycle may play out in the dynamics of the doughnut personality, that is, the interplay between the "dough" and the "bad jelly." It may be that hallucinations, such as the void in the sky experienced by Juan, or the persecutory voices commonly experienced by people suffering from schizophrenia may represent an attempt to externalize the unintegrated bad object representations. These are experienced by the individual suffering from schizophrenia as separate and terrifying, and yet they may also feel like they are controlled by these hallucinations. The escape to the megalomanic edge of the "dough" is an attempt to ward off and defend against these unintegrated aggressive object images or representations.

Replacement children

A child's being a "replacement child" (Cain & Cain, 1964; Green & Solnit, 1964; V. Volkan & Ast, 1997) can be another negative ingredient in the channel containing biological and psychological materials that gives birth to the child's mind. The mother "deposits" (V. Volkan, 2015b; V. Volkan et al., 2002) the mental representation of a lost person, such as a child who had died before this baby was born, in the baby's developing core infantile self. "Depositing" is closely related to the well-known concept of "identification" in childhood. But it is in some ways significantly different than identification. In "identification" the child is the primary active partner in taking in and assimilating object images and related ego and superego functions from another person. In "depositing," the "other," an adult person, is more active in pushing his or her specific self and internalized object images into the child's developing infantile core self. The adult uses the child, mostly unconsciously, as a reservoir for certain self and object images that belong to that adult. The experiences that created these mental images in the adult are not "accessible" to the child. Yet those mental images are deposited or pushed into the child, but without the experiential/contextual "framework" that created them.

The depositor gives the child certain ego tasks, mostly unconsciously, to protect and maintain what is deposited in this child. Obviously, not all replacement children develop pathological conditions, though they may have behavior and personality patterns that are affected. For example, the effects of being a replacement child can be seen in the psychology of the popular singer Elvis Presley, which has been covered elsewhere (K. Volkan, 1994).

The replacement child develops his or her own ego functions in dealing with what has been pushed into him or her. For example, the replacement child will be preoccupied with the task of integrating the deposited image with the rest of his or her self-representation. The child may or may not succeed in doing so. If the mother unconsciously gives psychological tasks to the child not to integrate what had been put in her or him with the rest of the developing self, the child's ego's ability to integrate opposite psychological units may be disturbed. The child's initial core self becomes a battleground and is flooded with "bad" affects. One adult person with schizophrenia had externalized her internalized battle to the external world. Her "favorite" locations were cemeteries where sometimes she would have, in her delusional states, fights with the residents of the cemetery.

Especially from the psychoanalytic studies of the Holocaust we also became aware that adults in a child's environment deposit the traumatized and/or distorted self and object images in the child's developing infantile core self (V. Volkan 2015a; V. Volkan et al., 2002). This process can also become poisonous. Obviously if the child himself or herself may face drastic actual traumas ranging from losses or separations (a mother's or mothering person's postpartum depression or death, or the adoption of the child for example) to various sexualized or murderous tortures such as a mother regularly using her newborn baby as a penis for her masturbatory activities or locking up the baby in a closet so that his crying will not disturb the adults.

Examples of such actual or mental tortures are many. For example, a patient of one of the authors (K. Volkan) exemplifies this. This patient was seemingly normal, and she was able to function independently. However, one day she watched a television documentary about kidnapping and was suddenly overwhelmed with panic. She subsequently had a psychotic break resulting in hospitalization. Over a period of months, she was able to relate her life history. It turned out she had been locked in a shed by her mother, who suffered from schizophrenia, from infancy until three years of age and taken out only temporarily. As will be related below, this type of experience can lead to the development of an infantile psychotic core that can later be enveloped by a "healthy" self-representation. However, the healthy self may be fragile and a triggering event my cause reactivation of the infantile psychotic self, which is what seemed to have happened in this case.

Sometimes actual traumas are not due to unsatisfactory mothering, but real circumstances that render the mother helpless through no fault of her own. One of the male patients was subjected to many lifesaving surgeries as a child, including being tied to a hospital bed while he was given injections. As an adult such traumas were reflected in his bizarre sexual delusions and activities; he would put a blade in women's vaginas (representing his receiving injections) in order to excite them. Interestingly, he would find women who wanted to experience his sadism.

Early drastic traumas lead to the child's "actualizations" of early unconscious fantasies. Typical unconscious fantasies concern themselves with body functions, early object relations, birth, death, pregnancy, siblings, sex, and family romance. Actualization of the unconscious fantasies occurs when the associated actual trauma is very severe or when a series of actual traumas are accumulated that interfere with "the usual restriction of fantasy only, or mostly, to the psychological realm" (V. Volkan & Ast, 2001, p. 569). Actualization of the unconscious fantasy causes confusion as the child tries to evaluate where the fantasy ends and reality begins (V. Volkan, 2004a). For example, a mother preserved the "accidentally" severed finger of her son Attis in a jar and kept the jar in his bedroom out in the open. The boy's unconscious fantasy that one day his body would unite with the separated finger was "actualized." The story of Attis's total treatment has previously been published (V. Volkan, 2015a).

What the mother did was a reflection of her anxiety, which was internalized by her son inflaming the "bad" affects in his infantile core self, making it impossible for him to have a normal separation–individuation, maintain a normal body image, and have normal reality testing. At an advanced age, the boy's unconscious fantasy about a "detachable penis" was experienced as real, even though it was in fact a delusion. This type of delusion may become literalized in cases of autocastration (Gössler et al., 2002; Gyuris, 2011). This form of self-mutilation can be a precursor to the onset of schizophrenia. While it has been hypothesized that the lowering of testosterone levels following castration may contribute to the development of schizophrenia, it is also possible psychodynamic factors come in to play in such cases (Duggal et al., 2002).

So far, an incomplete list of negative ingredients has been mentioned. These ingredients are ones that were observed frequently during many years of clinical practice. As mentioned above, most likely none of these ingredients alone can create an infantile psychotic self. In order to establish such a fragile core, some or many of these ingredients must be mingled together or may be influenced by the child's neuro-biological issues. When these negative ingredients are present, what emerges from the test tube is a fragile infantile core psychic organization, that is, the infantile psychotic self, or a "seed of madness." The infantile psychotic self is saturated with peak "bad" affects that are related to aggression. The differentiation, integration, and reality testing potentials of the ego associated with the infantile psychotic self are damaged. The infantile psychotic self contains tensions between the inability to differentiate self-images from object images and a corresponding "psychobiological push" for psychological maturation. Other tensions are due to the child's attempt to externalize fragmented but often fused self- and object images and the corresponding inter-nalization of the same.

Most importantly, there is a "hunger" for libidinal experiences, but this hunger is never satisfied. Utilizing its available ego functions, the infantile psychotic self, like the early computer game character Pac-Man, or the wendigo monster (which we will discuss later), is doomed to "eat up" anything in front of it, without finding any food that is nourishing. The infantile psychotic self's main ego function is internalization. But it also evacuates constantly what has been "eaten."

Therefore, its other main ego function is externalization. The terms internalization and externalization are used to separate these functions from more sophisticated introjection and projection mechanisms in which there is some fit between what is projected and the target and between what is introjected and the reality of the object before it is taken in. Such fits do not exist in the externalizations and internalizations in individuals suffering from schizophrenia (Novick & Kelly, 1970). At times even these primitive ego mechanisms are not functional. The infantile psychotic self simply fuses with objects, only to separate from them.

It is more practical not to tie the development of an infantile psychotic self to a specific time in babyhood or childhood. Its crystallization takes place during the early developmental years. In some cases, an infantile psychotic self is formed through regression that occurs during the later developmental years. For example, a severe trauma during the oedipal or latency phase, such as a traumatizing incestuous relationship, rape by a priest, or when a mother increasingly experiences her offspring as a "dead" replacement child during the same time period that corresponds to the age of the first child when he or she died, induces excessive "bad" affects that saturate the non-psychotic infantile self and turns it into a psychotic infantile self. This can be seen in refugee camps or other locations where lives have been turned upside down after wars and war-like conditions (V. Volkan, 1988, 2006, 2017). At such places it is possible to see severely regressed individuals. None of these people had developed a true adult schizophrenia unless their condition was incipient before their severe regressions occurred.

An infantile *non-psychotic* self is libidinally saturated. The ego functions associated with it begin to differentiate from corresponding object images and integrate and assimilate "bad" aggressively invested self-images without being saturated with aggression. If everything goes well, a non-psychotic infantile self evolves and slowly gives rise to a cohesive and differentiated self-representation and corresponding cohesive and differentiated object representation and forms more mature new ego functions.

CHAPTER 17

Fates of infantile psychotic selves

If a child develops a non-psychotic infantile self, which matures and determines the individual's functional personality organization, there is the possibility that a previously existing infantile psychotic self could shrink or disappear. The analogy to this shrinking is the calcification of a tuberculosis lesion in a child's lung that does not cause problems for the rest of that child's life. This shrinking or disappearing can be inferred when treatment succeeds in modifying and strengthening the self-representation of an adult with schizophrenia without structurally changing the person's psychotic core. At least it is a theoretical possibility that such a fate could befall someone who has an infantile psychotic self-structure. The second potential fate of an infantile psychotic self is the opposite of the first one. This time the infantile psychotic self does not shrink, and a functional non-psychotic infantile self does not evolve. Under such a situation, the child develops *childhood schizophrenia*.

The other fates involve the psychological process called *encapsulation* (D. Rosenfeld, 1992; H. Rosenfeld, 1965; Tustin, 2018; V. Volkan, 1976, 1995). It means that an infantile psychotic self, which is not "calcified," becomes "surrounded" by a healthier self-representation that is the end result of a non-psychotic infantile self. The ego functions associated with the enveloping healthier self-representation are constantly obliged to pay attention to the influence of the infantile psychotic self and keep it under control. If the "encapsulation" is only partial, the healthy self absorbs aspects of the infantile psychotic self but still controls it, becoming its "spokesperson." The end result is the development of a "psychotic personality organization."

Psychotic personality organization

While people who possess such a personality organization can, to a great extent, hold on to their reality testing during their daily lives, they are involved in various, bizarre and often secret (from other people) repetitious thinking and action patterns. Such patterns are in the service of finding a "fit" between the infantile psychotic self and the environment, so that adaptation to life will not induce tensions in these individuals. Furthermore, such patterns may reflect these individuals' unending attempts to replace the "bad" affects of the infantile psychotic self with "good" libidinal ones. While they exhibit a "normal" front, clinical observations of peculiar thinking and action patterns lead to the diagnosis of a *psychotic personally organization*. This is often diagnosed, not as schizophrenia proper but schizophreniform disorder, or schizotypal personality disorder.

A patient was able to go to law school and graduate, but her psychotic personality organization resulted in her staying home (her husband had enough money to support both of them) and constantly relate to dozens and dozens of cats with leukemia. Her personal world centered on the cats and a veterinarian who looked after the animals. Real world issues, such as what was going on in her neighborhood or in the greater world, were not interesting to her, even though she had reality testing ability. During treatment it became clear that the sick cats represented her infantile psychotic self (V. Volkan, 2005).

In order to find a "fit" between her infantile psychotic self and the external world, this patient underwent six reconstructive surgical operations in an attempt to make her face resemble that of a cat. It may be that people with an infantile psychotic self-structure are represented among those who hoard animals. Animals, such as cats, can symbolically represent the infantile psychotic self. Taking care of such animals may be an attempt to provide "good" mothering in order to create a healthier self-representation that is at least partially able to encapsulate the infantile psychotic self. This attempt may need to be repeated, necessitating the hoarding of animals (K. Volkan, 2021).

Sometimes an adult's effective encapsulating "envelope" suddenly develops a "crack" and aspects of the infantile psychotic self erupt through it, causing a kind of focalized bizarre behavior, which may be transient or recurring. This crack occurs when the individual's current environment suddenly and drastically changes and, in the individual's mind, becomes identical with the early childhood environment that played a significant role in the evolution of the infantile psychotic, and later encapsulated, self. It is possible to suggest that such individuals suffer from *focalized psychosis*. A description of the case of a respected physician, Martinez, illustrates this mental condition (V. Volkan, 1995).

Martinez, a psychiatrist, was in the fifth year of his analysis when his analyst's wife died and the analyst became depressed. Martinez knew about the wife's death, but in spite of this, he and his analyst never discussed the death or the analyst's response to it. Instead, some months after losing his wife, the analyst terminated his work with Martinez, stating that the analysis had been successful. Soon after this, Martinez developed a focalized delusion, which led to his involvement in some bizarre activities, including sucking the breasts of obese women patients who came to his office, although his reality testing in other areas was not at all affected.

It is beyond the purpose of this book to recount Martinez's symptoms, but when Martinez sought a new analytic treatment for his focalized psychosis, it became clear that a crack in the "envelope" that surrounded Martinez's infantile psychotic self had occurred when his first psychoanalytic environment seemed to him to be identical with the childhood environment in which his infantile psychotic self had first evolved. For the first eight months of his life, Martinez was cared for by a severely depressed mother who had thoughts of murdering her infant and killing herself. She finally committed suicide. Meanwhile, baby Martinez, who had developed an infantile psychotic self, was taken care of by a grandmother, and under the older woman's care he developed a healthier infantile self, which evolved and encapsulated the infantile psychotic self. Martinez's bizarre behavior reflected the infantile psychotic self's searching for libidinalizing objects, while not being able to hold on to them.

The adult psychotic self

Another outcome of the infantile psychotic self illustrates the development of schizophrenia in a teenager or young adult. It reflects the consequences of paralysis of ego functions associated with the "envelope" that surrounds the infantile psychotic self. These individuals experience organismic panic and lose their existing personality structure. They then develop, at least for a short while, the "doughnut personality." They reexperience original childhood attempts to control the "seed of madness." Frantic attempts to control the middle of the doughnut "calm down" when the changed personality crystallizes as an adult psychotic self.

In the case of a psychotic personality organization, the infantile non-psychotic self (the envelope) evolves slowly and absorbs part of the infantile psychotic self while managing to encapsulate the latter. It becomes the "spokesperson" of the infantile psychotic self while remaining capable in most areas to test reality and act as a bridge to the external world. In the development of adult schizophrenia, the healthier self that surrounds the infantile psychotic self becomes shuttered. Unlike the slow process that characterizes the encapsulation of the infantile psychotic self in someone who will have a psychotic personality organization, for the people who will develop adult schizophrenia, the envelope that replaces the shattered encapsulating healthier self develops quickly in order to stop their organismic panic. The enveloping part does not become a "spokesperson" for the infantile psychotic self; but *is* the "voice" of the infantile psychotic self. It is not a bridge between the infantile psychotic self and the external world. It totally, or nearly totally, absorbs the infantile psychotic self so that the infantile psychotic self faces the external world. The crystallization of the adult psychotic self further changes the personality and makes it appear megalomanic before the patient handles this change through various adaptations.

The psychoanalytic techniques utilized for the treatment of adults with schizophrenia have been covered elsewhere and include a description of the *total* treatment processes illustrating these techniques (V. Volkan, 1976, 1995, 2015a). The concept of the adult psychotic self informs us about the major resistance to getting well that exists among patients with schizophrenia: They hold on to their adult psychotic selves in order to avoid experiencing another terror, an organismic panic. The psychoanalytic treatment that aims to make a structural change in the patient's internal world first needs to prepare the patient for experiencing a therapeutic organismic panic in order to help them to go through another personality change, this time a healthier one. A most detailed description of dealing with a therapeutic organismic panic and decomposition of an adult psychotic self is drawn from the treatment of Jane whose total analysis has been described in detail (V. Volkan, 1995) and to whose case we will refer again in Chapter 21 and 23.

Some adults are called individuals with schizophrenia because they experienced childhood schizophrenia, which has continued in modified ways into adulthood. This chapter illustrates a theory about the etiology of adult schizophrenia, which appears in teenagers or young adults who seemed to have no major psychological problems until their schizophrenia develops. An adult suffering from schizophrenia is regressed due to the reappearance of an already existent, previously covered over (encapsulated) fragile core (an infantile psychotic self) and its re-encapsulation by a self that becomes the voice of this core. It is suggested that psychoanalysts continue to examine the internal worlds of adults with schizophrenia or related conditions in order not to deprive ourselves of obtaining further data on primitive mental states and psychoanalytically informed techniques to improve or cure them. Insights emerging from this examination may be relevant for some who suffer from chronic and/or medicated schizophrenia, who in the past would not have been considered candidates for psychotherapy.

Part III

Psychoanalytic approaches to treating schizophrenia

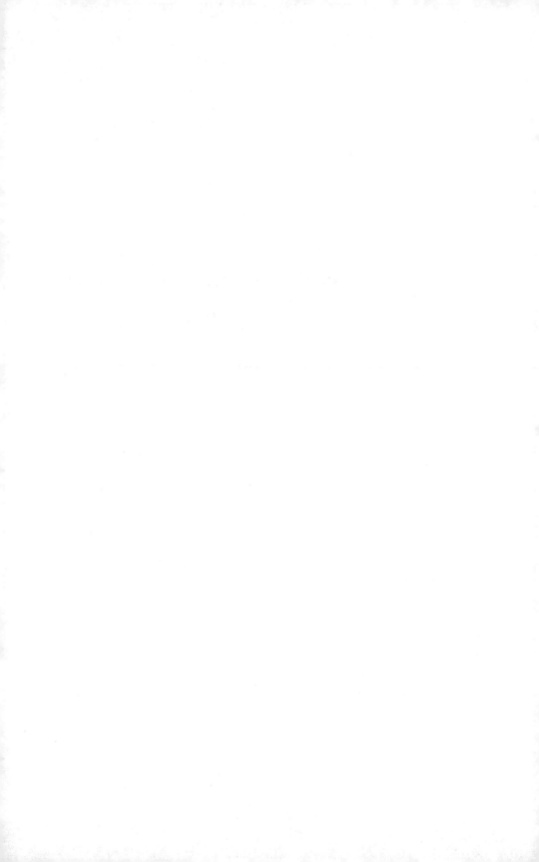

Psychodynamic approaches to treating schizophrenia

Sigmund Freud believed that psychoanalysis could not be successfully used with patients suffering from schizophrenia, but that has not stopped psychodynamic psychotherapists from trying to work with patients suffering from this disorder over the years. There are many examples of psychodynamic treatments with patients suffering from schizophrenia with some important examples presented below.

Freud's most famous follower, until he broke off to form his own form of analysis, Carl Jung, began his career treating patients with schizophrenia and later made valuable efforts to understand the symbolism that appeared in psychotic symptoms (Jung, 1925). Other of Freud's followers also attempted to at least understand schizophrenia following Freud's principles (Ferenczi & Jones, 1916). Charles Tidd (1937) reported the successful psychoanalytic treatment of a patient we might now label as schizotypal. He went on to report on the use of psychoanalytic treatment with patients suffering from schizophrenia that had undergone shock (convulsive) therapies (Tidd, 1938). Benjamin Weininger (1938) recommended modification of psychoanalytic technique to be more active during acute psychosis. Frieda Fromm-Reichmann (1939) maintained that psychoanalysts could develop and maintain workable relationships with patients suffering from schizophrenia and that successful psychotherapy requires understanding a different kind of transference phenomena. Ronald Fairbairn (1952), who was one of the principal figures in the British object relations school of psychoanalysis, proposed revisions to Freud's original libido theory in terms of the development of object relations. He also modified psychoanalytic techniques when working with patients suffering from schizophrenia. In the 1950s French psychoanalyst Gisela Pankow developed a technique she called dynamic structuring that combined working with clay, psychoanalysis, and phenomenological therapy to help patients suffering from schizo-phrenia (Valon, 2020). More modern analytic-based therapies have built on Pankow's work (Bonnigal-Katz, 2019). By the 1970s Harold Searles (1986) greatly contributed to the psychoanalytic understanding of schizophrenia. He proposed a more direct analytic approach to working with patients suffering from schizophrenia. More recently David Downing and John Mills (2018) have compiled evidence-based psychodynamic approaches to treatment for individuals suffering from schizophrenia in outpatient settings.

These are just some of the psychoanalytic clinicians who have worked with patients suffering from schizophrenia over the last 100 years. Psychodynamic approaches to treating schizophrenia have waxed and waned over time. An influential but deeply flawed study demonstrating that antipsychotic medication had as good results as analytic treatment had a huge negative impact on the use of psychody-namic therapies with patients suffering from schizophrenia (May, 1968). However, the psychoanalytic treatment in the study was provided by very poorly trained resident physicians and was clearly not up to the level of a properly trained analyst or psychodynamic therapist. Nevertheless, after the study was published, interest in using psycho-dynamic-related treatment for schizophrenia dropped precipitously (Stone, 1999). Other past reviews have suggested the negative effects of psychodynamic treatment of patients suffering from schizophrenia (Mueser & Berenbaum, 1990).

Nevertheless, there are some modern psychodynamic therapists and analysts who have done psychotherapy or even a modified form of psychoanalysis with psychotic patients with good success (Gibbs, 2007;

Giovachinni & Boyer, 1980; Gottdiener, 2006; Grotstein, 2001, 2003; Kortegaard, 1993; V. Volkan, 1995, 2015b).

As will be explored below, there is a good deal of evidence that a psychodynamic approach can be useful; possibly even with long-term patients in an inpatient setting (Davenport et al., 2000). It is also thought that a psychodynamic understanding of schizophrenia can help improve treatment even when the treatment itself is not psycho-dynamic (Kline et al., 1992). Richard Lucas (2003) suggests that psychodynamic approaches to treatment give clinicians a way in which to symbolically understand and communicate with their patients suffering from schizophrenia in a way that can help them make sense of their situation. As will be discussed, understanding of symbolic communication can lead to a transferential therapeutic relationship that has great potential in helping and even curing some types of people suffering from schizophrenia.

Wilfried Eecke (2019) advocates using a Lacanian form of treatment with patients suffering from schizophrenia. This approach follows Lacan's idea that people with schizophrenia are unable to integrate a "third" in their personalities. The person suffering from schizo-phrenia has a psychic structure that is a dyad between the infant and an omnipotent mother. An ego-structuring technique is used to let such people perceive themselves outside of this dyad and allow them to discover themselves as a separate individual.

It is interesting to note from the studies cited above that much of the work using psychodynamic approaches to working with patients suffering from schizophrenia is being done outside of the United States. France in particular has been pioneering psychoanalytic based therapies for use with people suffering from schizophrenia (Kapsambelis, 2019).

Most psychodynamic approaches to the treatment of schizophrenia assume that psychotic processes develop in early childhood and are related to either a withdrawal from the world or an inability to separate from being psychically fused with a mother figure (De Masi, 2020). This may be due to pathological neurobiology, structural changes in the brain, and/or pathogenic parenting.

One of the authors of this book, Vamık Volkan, has extensive experience conducting psychoanalysis with people who have psychotic self-organization. His work suggests that psychoanalysis can be used to help the patient modify the infantile psychotic self and achieve separation–individuation. This approach to understanding schizophrenia can be considered as the most comprehensive to come out of psychoanalysis. In Chapter 20 we will go into depth about how he has applied an object relations approach to treating people suffering from schizophrenia.

CHAPTER 19

Psychoanalytic treatment of adults suffering from schizophrenia

It goes without saying that the treatment of adults suffering from schizophrenia is a difficult process. At the present time most therapeutic attempts to treat them include medication as well as a combination of approaches such as applied behavior analysis, various psychotherapies, and interventions with family members.

Such approaches range from sophisticated understanding of the psychodynamics of the patients' internal worlds, to completely ignoring such psychodynamics. Often medications are used, especially in the USA, to satisfy the requirements of insurance coverage and protect the caregivers from legal suits. There have been occasions when the caregivers were sued by the patient's relatives whose lawyers charged that, by not giving antipsychotic drugs to the patient, the therapist was responsible for improper treatment. On the other hand, there have been some impressive examples of sophisticated combinations of various treatment approaches.

One example of this comes from Finland where Yrjö Alanen (1993) created a method called "need-adapted treatment." For a most recent success report of this method, see Schulmann, 2004. Another example comes from the Austen Riggs Center in Massachusetts, USA, which has been in continuous operation since the early 1900s. This is one of the last elite private hospitals for serious mental illness where patients can receive intensive long-term psychotherapy. Patients at Austen Riggs are not committed to the hospital but enter voluntarily and may leave at any time. The treatment modality at Austen Riggs in general follows the principle of psychodynamic psychopharmacology. Most patients receive medication, including those who are diagnosed as suffering from schizophrenia, but also receive psychoanalytically oriented psychotherapy four times a week as well as participate in certain very specific types of community activities. The psychodynamic psychopharmacology pioneered at Austen Riggs has recently gained empirical support. Angela Iannitelli and her colleagues (Iannitelli et al., 2019), in a review of studies examining combined pharmacological and psychoanalytic treatments for schizophrenia, found that these treatment modalities can be used in combination to great effect.

This review will *only* focus on certain aspects of psychoanalytic treatment of adults suffering from schizophrenia and the metapsychological explanations of these treatments. This brings up an important first question: Which adults suffering from schizophrenia are suitable for a psychoanalytic approach to their treatment? It is important to note that those adults suffering from schizophrenia who became ill because of an extreme burden of genetic/biological/structural factors are not likely to be suitable for a psychoanalytic approach. It is essential to clearly mention this because critiques of psychoanalysis and psychoanalytic-derived therapies for people suffering from schizophrenia are often centered on the failure of these therapies to successfully treat *all* people suffering from schizophrenia (Willick, 2001). The case being made here is that *some* individuals suffering from schizophrenia are amenable to psychoanalytic based treatments, but not all. More individuals suffering from schizophrenia may be suitable for a combined psychoanalytic therapy plus medication approach to treatment.

It is difficult, but not impossible, to measure the weight of the genetic/biological factors against that of experiential disturbances/traumas of childhood. It is expected that advances in epigenetics will begin to decode these associations (Adam & Harwell, 2020; Colangeli, 2020; Gong & Xu, 2017; J.-Y. Hwang et al., 2017; Leuzinger-Bohleber, 2016; Smigielski et al., 2020; Weigel & Scharbert, 2016). There is, however, still much confounding among the factors that could possibly induce schizophrenia in a human being. Clearly, methods for distinguishing who among those that suffer from schizophrenia could benefit from psychoanalytic treatment and psychoanalytic treatment combined with other treatment modalities needs further research. Thus, the cases and theory presented here in support of the idea that psychoanalytic therapy could be helpful to some patients suffering from schizophrenia is preliminary. Further information, such as that provided by Fred Levin (2011) and, of course, improvements in our ability to measure the link between "mind" and "brain," are needed. However, since the brain changes when modifications are made in the mind, the inclusion of genetic/biological issues in the genesis of adult schizophrenia should not stop us from understanding and treating these patients psychoanalytically.

The emerging and exciting findings in neuropsychoanalysis will eventually allow us to more closely correlate genetic, biological, and structural changes in the brain to the specific stages of development of schizophrenia (Johnson & Flores Mosri, 2016; Marini et al., 2016). For instance, Anatolia Salone and her colleagues (2016) describe possible neurological correlates to self-structures and processes as well as ego functions in patients suffering from schizophrenia. While this work is in its infancy it holds great promise. It would be good to know which people suffering from schizophrenia have a predominantly organic/genetic etiology vs. those who lean towards more psychological origins of the disease. Quick differential diagnosis between these origins of schizophrenia could identify a subset of people suffering from schizophrenia who would be most likely to benefit from intensive psychotherapy or psychoanalysis. Research such as the study cited above by Philippe Conus and associates (2017) may indicate some characteristics that could be a good starting point for determining that patients suffering from schizophrenia may obtain the greatest benefit from psychotherapeutic approaches to treatment.

The above statements notwithstanding, there are some things we do know. The level of "bizarreness" in the clinical picture presented, as clinical experience shows, is not a good criterion for predicting the outcome of a long-term psychoanalytic approach. For example, a twenty-two-year-old woman had hallucinations, delusions, and painted her hospital room with and ate her feces. This young woman, in the long run, provided an example of a successfully treated adult suffering from schizophrenia by a psychoanalytic approach with on and off hospitalizations—without receiving any medication.

Lastly, one has to take into consideration the *chronicity* of the psychotic adult self. Harold Searles (1961) in a contribution now considered a classic, described phases of the patient/therapist interactions in the treatment of adults suffering from schizophrenia. His first phase dealt with the "chronic" existence of the psychotic adult self. Vamık Volkan's analytic experiences working with such individuals (1964, 1976, 1986, 1990, 1995, 2015a), with the exception of two individuals, were with adults suffering from schizophrenia whose psychotic adult selves had not become chronic. By "chronicity" we are referring to the severe crystal-lization of the structure of the psychotic adult self, and not necessarily to the number of years that passed since the individual experienced his or her terror (organismic panic).

Searles called his first phase of treatment of individuals suffering from chronic schizophrenia the "out of contact" phase. Vamık Volkan reports that all the adult patients with whom he worked psychoanalyti-cally, except the two, were "in contact" with the analyst from the very beginning. This contact being defined by the patient's ability to take his image (as they experienced it) into their fusing–disconnecting or internalization–externalization cycles (the nature of these cycles will be described presently). This may be another key point for discovering which patients suffering from schizophrenia will be able to benefit from psychotherapy or psychoanalysis.

Another important point when considering psychoanalytic treatment with people suffering from schizophrenia is that psychoanalysts and psychotherapists vary in their ability and potential for regression in the service of their patients (Olinick, 1980). Typically, a psychoanalyst/psychotherapist's own personal therapeutic experience regress them only to neurotic levels and not to psychotic levels. Therefore, we can safely assume that many psychoanalysts do not have experiences in which they visit or stay for any length of time in severely regressed states, and therefore they do not particularly have an interest in working with severely regressed individuals. To do so would necessitate their own regression in the service of their patients in order to meet them at their severely regressed states. They may also subscribe to a theoretical position that working at severely regressed states is impossible, if not detrimental for the patient.

There may be a role for talent and experience here. Some therapists will naturally have more of a talent for regression in the service of their patients, while others will have a difficult and perhaps frightening experience trying to do this. It is likely the therapists' own life history and experiences will determine this.

We are not suggesting that those clinicians who choose to work with adults who suffer from schizophrenia suffer from regressive psychopathology themselves. For example, one of this book's authors' cultural background—having a grandfather who threshed wheat by sitting on a wooden plank that had sharp stones under it, and that was pulled by cows or donkeys, and also having children who are sophisticated in their use of most advanced technological instruments—has made it rather easy for him to travel, psychologically speaking, from the stone age to the computer age. The other author began his career working and practically living with individuals suffering from schizophrenia in a residential facility for a number of years, as well as delving into a number of meditative practices that include regression and introjective–projective mental exercises (K. Volkan, 2013). These types of experiences may make it more comfortable to work with individuals suffering from schizophrenia and help to empathize with their state of mind. Non-interpretive creative dreamwork such as "embodied imagination" created by psychoanalyst Robert Bosnak (1996, 2007) provides a way for psychotherapists to learn to engage with deep unconscious and chaotic imagery while maintaining some conscious awareness. The ability to practice with this "dual consciousness" could be useful in working with people suffering from schizophrenia.

Another consideration that should also be noted is that many mental health professionals have not had much, if any, experience working with individuals suffering from schizophrenia. Those mental health professionals who have worked with people suffering from schizophrenia are likely to have focused on medication management (psychiatrists) or behavioral treatment (non-MD clinicians). It is likely that neither professional training nor clinical experience has included consideration of the developmental psychodynamics of individuals suffering from schizophrenia.

Two factors may give clues to psychoanalysts and psychothera-pists who are interested in treating patients with psychotic adult selves as described here and about the appropriateness of taking such individuals into psychodynamic treatment. The first one refers to the therapist's empathic understanding of the meaning of the patient's bizarre symptoms during the diagnostic work. For example, Sanford, a nineteen-year-old man diagnosed with schizophrenia often cut himself and examined his blood. He believed that his blood had different colors at different times, as he experienced himself as different individuals. During the diagnostic interview it became clear that he was searching for "true blood" and "true identity." When he mentioned he was an adopted child, his symptom started to make sense.

The second factor is how the patient reacts when the analyst makes a remark about the patient's initial "eating" (internalization) of the analyst's image. An adult who suffers from schizophrenia who is not in an "out of contact" (Searles, 1961) state (we also believe that this state never totally dominates the patient's relatedness to the other) will relate to the therapist during the diagnostic interviews through fusing–disconnecting or internalization–externalization cycles. Such individuals will fuse their perceived self-images with the image of the therapist and behave as if the two persons are one, and after a while they will separate the two images. This cycle will continue. Or the patient will keep his or her image within its own border, however fragile it may be, but take in the analyst's image ("eat" it) and after a while "spit it out." Again, the cycle will continue. In our experience, if the patient reacts "positively" to the therapist's initial explanation of being included in such cycles, this is a good indication for taking such an individual into psychoanalytic treatment.

A patient suffering from schizophrenia heard that his analyst (Vamık Volkan) was of Turkish origin. He ate a *turkey dinner* before coming to see him the next morning. When he met his analyst, he reported this and then looked very scared and turned pale. It was understood that for him a bird/turkey was not a symbol, but a protosymbol (Werner & Kaplan, 1984). The bird/turkey was not a symbol of the analyst; it *was* the analyst. Therefore, it was possible to sense that for this man, at this hour, the analyst should not exist. Or the analyst was only a scary ghost. The analyst responded to him by saying calmly that what he ate was a bird/turkey. He added that he was a man who was connected with the country Turkey and that he continued to exist in the external world after the patient had eaten his dinner. But that the analyst wanted him to know that he understood the reason for the patient's "anxiety"—his mixing the bird/turkey with the analyst and the analyst's connection with Turkey. The patient then said nothing, but briefly showed a big—and it might be said, a warm—smile. The analyst sensed that he had made an empathic connection with the patient. It should be said here that in the analyst's response to the patient turning pale, he was following the classical dictum for psychoanalytic treatment: Start from the surface and go slowly deeper. For a patient like this man, the surface *is* the material that would have been considered "deep" if he were functioning on a neurotic level.

The first dominant resistance of adults suffering from schizophrenia to getting well—that is, their giving up their adult psychotic selves—is their stubborn attempt to protect themselves from experiencing another terror (organismic panic). For these individuals, the original organismic panic occurred when their then-existing healthier selves that enveloped their infantile psychotic selves were shuttered and the ego functions associated with their healthier selves were paralyzed. After developing their adult psychotic selves and after escaping their original organismic panic, such individuals will hold onto their adult psychotic selves, their new but psychotic identities, as if their life depended on them—this in order not to experience another internal "star explosion" loss of identity. Nevertheless, in order for them to get well (by "getting well" we are referring to such individuals making an internal structural change in their psychic organizations and not a seemingly better adjustment to their psychotic state) they have to experience once more an organismic panic as their adult psychotic selves are crushed and replaced by healthier selves. The organismic panic is a response to losing existing identity. For these individuals, such an internal change, even the one that will lead to a positive outcome, is not accompanied by average anxiety, but by an "emotional flooding" (V. Volkan, 1976).

Accordingly, if the treatment approach to an adult suffering from schizophrenia is not simply supportive but also psychoanalytic, these patients need to be prepared to experience an emotional flooding (organismic panic) within their psychotic transference to the analyst or therapist. The patients prepare themselves for this drastic experience by borrowing ego functions from their analysts and then identifying with them.

Before proceeding further, we would like to make clear that we are *not* presenting a comprehensive list of technical maneuvers for the psychoanalytic psychotherapy of adult patients suffering from schizophrenia. This is covered in detail elsewhere (V. Volkan, 1976, 1981, 1990, 1995, 2015a). Rather, our aim is to illustrate that such patients' various types of internalizations of and/or identifications with their therapists and their ego functions are absolutely necessary to their making internal structural changes in the process of getting well. By "internalization" we are referring to *an activity* whereby, when an individual's self-representation, which is to some extent differentiated and separated from the images of objects, takes in an object image. On the other hand, "identification" is *a state of affairs* (Fuchs, 1937) whereby the internalized object image is unconsciously absorbed into an individual's self-representation.

More modern ideas about identification focus on an individual's taking in and absorbing their *experiences* with the object in order to enrich their sense of self and strengthen existing ego functions and/or develop new ones. Accordingly, Stanley Greenspan (1990) suggested that we no longer use the term "identification" that refers to its classic meaning. We continue to use it since it is clinically very useful. Both internalization and identification processes in people suffering from schizophrenia are accompanied by cannibalistic incorporative fantasies clearly reflecting the psychological processes mentioned above. A more primitive phenomenon than internalization is "fusing" (in the literature the term "merging" is sometimes used) one's self-representation with the object image without the act of internalization that led to quick identifications. Such identifications are not stable and are temporary.

CHAPTER 20

Fusing–disconnecting and internalization–externalization cycles

The ego functions of the psychotic adult self, as the "voice" of the infantile psychotic self, are centered upon maintaining primitive object relations: to be engaged with object images in a fusing–disconnecting and/or an internalization–externalization cycle. The patient is *object hungry*. An attempt is made to collect "good" images in order to libidinalize the infantile and adult psychotic selves, but the patient also collects "bad" objects under the influence of repetition-compulsion, and certainly in the patients' experience what is "eaten" as good might easily turn out to be bad. Thus, such adults suffering from schizophrenia, while obliged to fuse with or take in object images, are also obliged to omnipotently control such images when they appear to be located in external objects. These patients are therefore both dependent on external objects and preoccupied with putting a buffer between themselves and external objects. This may result in a confusing clinical picture.

Without the ability to stabilize the collection of "good" objects, the patient's ego's ability to integrate "good" and "bad" object images is deficient. Such patients, as we discussed earlier, also exhibit a splitting mechanism that keeps "good" and "bad" object images separate and sometimes fragmented. Patients with borderline personality organization have mastered the utilization of splitting. But an adult schizophrenic patient's splitting mechanism is not stable.

When adults suffering from schizophrenia begin psychoanalytic treatment, inevitably and often right away, they will include their analyst's images, as they perceive them, in fusing–disconnecting and/ or internalization–externalization cycles. Kleinian oriented therapists of today who treat adults suffering from schizophrenia psychoanalyti-cally frequently refer to the concept of "projective identification" (Klein, 1946) to explain the nature of such patients' major relationships with their therapists (Schulmann, 2004). Hanna Segal (1988), a key follower of Klein, described projective identification as follows: "Parts of the self and internal objects are split off and projected into the external object, which then becomes possessed by, controlled and identified with the projected parts" (p. 27).

It is preferable to speak about an internalization–externalization cycle, which may describe what is observed among people suffering from schizophrenia in a more graphic way. In adults suffering from schizophrenia, especially in acute cases, when what is externalized boomerangs back into the patient's self-representation, it seldom leads to a stable identification, but is quickly externalized once again. But the term internalization–externalization cycle should also cover the Kleinian concept of projective identification as it appears in the transference–countertransference relationship between the patient and the analyst.

Initially the analyst's task is *not* to interpret why the patients are stuck in this type of object relations, but to be experientially involved in such cycles while keeping their observing and analyzing functions intact. The analyst can explain the nature of the patient's object relations and make such experiences describable through word symbols. The aim is to initiate a process that will help the patient retain internalized good object images as identifications that can libidinalize the infantile and adult psychotic selves. As Norman Cameron (1961) observed, for adults suffering from schizophrenia it is possible "to 'introject' massively with archaic completeness in adulthood and then be able to assimilate the new introject as an infant might, so that it disappears as such, but some of its properties do not" (p. 93).

A case of one of the authors (Vamık Volkan) demonstrates how the internalization–externalization cycle can be observed and worked with:

> After seeing my name on my office door, a young man suffering from schizophrenia, Ricky, believed that I was German. During his initial session with me he made sucking sounds. When I showed my curiosity about it, he reported that he was drinking German wine (my image was fused with his early mother image whom he had named "Hitler" because he had experienced his mother as intruding upon his developing autonomy). I knew that the German wine Ricky was "drinking" was "bad," because of his facial expressions. I told him that I am Turkish, not German. He anxiously asked me if Turks make wine too. I answered "Yes." He then asked if Turks make sweet or sour wine. I said "Both" and added, "You have a choice. Pick either one." He chose the "sweet" Turkish wine and would continue to "drink" me for many sessions to come until I became sour Turkish wine and then sweet Turkish wine and the cycle continued.
>
> During my interaction with Ricky described above I first added a "reality" by informing him that I am Turkish. By telling him that Turks had sweet and sour wines, I gave him "good" and "bad" targets for externalizations. I focused on the experience between us. I did not interpret his reasons for calling his mother "Hitler" and his initially fusing my image with hers. Even if I interpreted such things, most likely he would not "hear" me.
>
> After drinking sweet Turkish wine during his sessions for many months Ricky developed an internal voice with a Turkish accent, which would tell him what to do. But another internal voice also developed with a German accent telling Ricky not to listen to the first voice.
>
> When my internalized object image began competing with his "Hitler mother" image and Ricky became flustered, I told him that there was no rush to choose between the two voices. Recalling that he had experienced an internal voice speaking with a German accent in the past and knowing that he had devoured books about the Nazis in order to learn about them, I suggested that the voice with the Turkish accent was rather new to him. I added that surely, he was not yet sure if this Turkish voice would be helpful to him. He should take his time to test and get to know this new voice.

Only in the second year of his treatment I learned that Ricky was reading history books about Turks. Learning that Turks had a reputation as "terrible" warmongers, he put a buffer between us. During his sessions he would whistle so that my voice would not be heard (would not be introjected through his ears). So, I asked him out loud to stop whistling and when he did, I said that he was free to tell me when he perceived me as a scary person and that I had no intention of killing him. The whistling slowly stopped and then I noticed his using my image as a libidinalizing object. I became his "Turkish delight" who taught him how to test reality.

Ricky was born with a deformed hand. His mother denied his deformity. For example, when Ricky was a small child his mother would buy him rings for his birthdays. None of these rings would fit his deformed ring finger. Ricky could not "learn" from his mother what was real. Whenever I was his "Turkish delight" he would raise issues during our sessions and ask me about the realities of such issues. Some of these were simple things: Did I know the exact distance between Charlottesville and Washington? At first, I replied directly and told him the "truth." Then I asked him to find out the answers so that he could develop his autonomy. When he resisted this, I dealt with the resistance telling him, for example, that if he figured out the distance between Charlottesville and Washington by himself and reported it to me, I would still be around and not leave him. In fact, we could then experience a relationship between two knowledgeable individuals. This in fact, might be exciting and pleasurable.

At times Ricky would sexualize his "eating" a Turkish delight and behave as if he were submitting to me sexually. At this time the interaction between us was in the service of his collecting object images that would libidinalize his core. Knowing this I would deal with his anxiety and bewilderment for sexual submission by joining his "reaching up," which was a resistance and for example telling him that "good things" can come from both women and men. After Ricky had maintained my libidinalizing Turkish image long enough, he moved up to identify with more mature and sophisticated analyst functions.

What is important is to follow what patients do with the analyst's introjected image and how, in the long run, the analyst's introjected image becomes libidinalizing for the patient's adult and, by extension, infantile psychotic self (in Ricky's case how he would maintain sweet Turkish wine). When the internalization of the analyst's image becomes stable, a competition between the introjected analyst image and already existing archaic images often appear (Abse & Ewing, 1960). The analyst uses explanations that describe and verbalize the nature of this competition. The analyst should not force a positive outcome concerning internalizations but wait for the natural evolution of an internalization–externalization cycle and continue to verbalize and explain the conflicts that arise during this process.

During the initial phase of treatment (which sometimes takes years) the transference of adults who suffer from schizophrenia is dominated by their fusing–disconnecting and internalization–externalization cycles that is the essence of a psychotic transference. Sometimes such a patient slows down these cycles and concentrates intensively on the therapist as an object of his or her libidinal or aggressive targeting. The therapist has to deal with such situations.

In the second year of her analysis twenty-two-year-old Lilian's understanding and sensing of her internalization–externalization cycles improved greatly and slowed down. Her male therapist whom Vamık Volkan was supervising sensed that his patient had a fear of losing her usual way of behaving. Most likely as a defense against facing this "loss," the patient exhibited an eroticized psychotic trans-ference. After starting her sessions, she started to pull her dress up to her belly and show her legs and underwear to her therapist. While in her therapist's office she also stated that she soon might also take off her underwear. In a supervisory hour the therapist was reminded that he was also a spokesperson of "realities." In his next session with Lilian, the therapist told her that he wanted to speak first. Gently, he made the following remarks:

> I have some ideas about why you pulled your dress up and showed me your legs during recent sessions. It is crucial that I share my ideas about this with you *now*. Parents sometimes show their love by holding their infants and small babies while the little ones are not fully dressed. One of the reasons why you want to undress before me is a wish to repeat such a caretaker-small baby relationship with me. But in reality, you are no longer a baby. In reality, you and

I are observing and learning about your childhood experiences together by putting your thoughts, feelings, and recollections into words. And there is another reality. No one taught me to conduct therapy while my patient is showing me her underwear. I want you to stop showing me your legs up to your hips by pulling your dress up. If you do so, the session will end at that moment. I am telling you this not as a rejection of you, but as an expression of my wish to remain as your therapist and allowing us to continue to work. And I want to continue to work with you.

It was difficult for the therapist and his supervisor to know fully if Lilian understood her therapist's explanation. However, she responded positively to his being a spokesperson of realities.

For a patient with a neurotic personality organization, the analyst is not a full reincarnation of archaic objects (a transference figure). Indeed, the analyst will become a transference figure but, as an empathetic model for curiosity about the patient's internal world, eventually he or she will also become a different unique therapeutic figure called by various names, such as *new object, developmental object,* or *analytic introject*—for examples see Baker, 1993; Cameron, 1961; Chused, 1982; Giovacchini, 1972; Kernberg, 1975; Loewald, 1960; Tähkä, 1993; V. D. Volkan, 1976, 2010, 2021. The analyst's newness does not refer to his or her social existence in the real world but depends on the analyst being an object (and its representation) not hitherto encountered. The patient's interaction with a "new object" is akin to a nurturing child–mother relationship (Ekstein, 1966; Rapaport, 1951). Patients with schizophrenia initially perceive the analyst's images as totally libidinized or totally aggressively saturated, later as integrated with different ego and superego functions. In successful treatments they also experience the analyst image as a "new object." Lilian's therapist was careful not to sound as if he was ordering her to do this or that, or turning the analytic introject into a severe superego.

Another of Vamık Volkan's cases exemplifies how one of his patients perceived him as totally dangerous and how he dealt with this situation:

Lisa at one time contaminated me with her uncaring mother's "bad" archaic object image. For many sessions I felt that she was "out of contact." Then one day she "allowed" me to notice that at the beginning of her sessions she would put a candy called a Lifesaver in her mouth and keep it there hidden during the sessions. Thus, I could not go into her body (representing her existing psychotic adult self) as a "bad" object through her mouth. I told her that when she felt safe, she could stop this ritual and have a relationship with me without a buffer. I suggested that she was free to tell me if our experience without a buffer might be scary for her. If this was the case, I was always willing to go at her pace. Soon after this exchange Lisa began experimenting with not putting a Lifesaver into her mouth.

Also, it is more urgent to deal with the patient's disturbing reactions to fusing with or internalizing "bad" object images rather than their "bad" externalizations. When "bad" externalizations are placed steadily upon the analyst, the analyst notices this continuing externalization and his or her counterresponse. The trained psychoanalyst will tolerate this situation for an appropriate time without trying to send back the patient's externalized images prematurely. At such times analysts are required to notice their counter response (countertransference) and tolerate such externalizations for an appropriate time without trying to send them back right away to the patient. Furthermore, analysts need to pay attention to events that are seemingly outside of the patient's psychotic transference toward the analyst. While working with a neurotic patient, analysts may decide to pay attention only—or primarily—to transference manifestations and not get too easily involved in the extra-transference issues. At the initial phase of the analytic treatment of adults suffering from schizophrenia, some extra-transference events induce intense affects in such patients and interfere with the therapeutic process. Analysts need to pay attention to them instead of waiting for a similar situation to evolve in the transference.

Sanford, the young man mentioned above who used to cut himself and check on the color of his blood, met a couple and, in his delusional state, believed that they were his biological parents. He approached them but they thought he was "crazy" and they treated him badly. After this, Sanford came to his sessions in a panic-stricken state, mimicking the couple's gestures and facial expressions. Sanford was told that he was disappointed in the couple and his feeling of disappointment was strong enough to link him to them. It was pointed out that often our having bad feelings connects us with those who are targets of such feelings. More importantly, Sanford was directed to tell and retell his encounter with the couple. This brought a great deal of reality to the actual event of the encounter, and he began to separate his image from the image of the couple.

CHAPTER 21

Development of a steady identification with the "good" analyst

Interestingly the patient's steady identification with the "good" image of the analyst, an image saturated with libidinal investments, leads to another organismic panic, but this experience of emotional flooding is *therapeutic*, as Vamık Volkan describes:

> During her ten—twelve initial months of treatment with me, Jane, a twenty-one-year-old college student, primarily experienced my images as "bad," and my "bad" image was involved in her internalization–externalization cycle. Both of us tolerated this. Then I noticed her regarding me steadily as a new "good" object. Sitting in front of me she would ask me to turn this or that way and move into or away from the light. I did not move and said nothing, basically because I did not understand what was going on. She explained that she was taking my picture by blinking her eyes. Then I could clearly observe her becoming a camera and her blinking eyes like the shutter of a camera. When she left my presence, she went to a dark room and mentally developed my picture (projecting it onto the external world but keeping it near her). This behavior went on for some months. Meanwhile we were able to define my function for her as a "good" object. As a child she could not depend on her mother who was depressed due

to losing Jane's sister, who died at the age of three, when Jane was one and a half. Neither could Jane depend on her father's image. By "losing" his wife to depression, he had turned to Jane and made her his target for incestuous activities. I was a new "good" object image that could help Jane develop "basic trust." (Erikson, 1950)

When the adult suffering from schizophrenia absorbs the introjected "good" analyst image in a stable fashion—experience has demonstrated that this usually happens in the second year of a four-times-a week psychoanalytic treatment—the patient lets go of the adult psychotic self. Losing existing identity ushers in another organismic panic. Instead of feeling a signal anxiety concerning the danger of an internal loss, the patient becomes emotionally flooded with aggressive or libidinal affects. Before the lost psychotic self is replaced by a healthier one, the patient once more will feel as if he or she is a monster or an angel. What is interesting is that the patient's experience of the second organismic panic is usually contained. It happens during a session or a few consequent sessions instead of in a prolonged generalized way in the external world.

Typically, patients begin their experiences of emotional flooding by recalling real or fantasized events one after another that support the same emotion. Soon the recalled emotion peaks. The patient screams or laughs uncontrollably. In 1976 Vamık Volkan wrote about how patients describe undergoing a "metamorphosis" during the experience, "becoming monstrous or diabolical when the signal affects were replaced by primal affects closely related to the aggressive drive. If the primal affect was close to the libidinal drive, however, there was another kind of change, the kind reflected in poetry or prose when a lover tells his beloved, '… I love you so much that I am a new person …' In this state, the representation of the affect becomes the patient's perceived self" (p. 185).

After the patient and the analyst tolerate the second organismic panic, the patient begins to experience signal anxiety when perceiving a psychological danger. This is a sign indicating that a healthier self has replaced the psychotic adult self and now envelopes—much more effectively than the adult psychotic self—the infantile psychotic self. According to Vamık Volkan, when he first started working intensively with adults suffering from schizophrenia whose conditions had not become chronic, he would ask patients to use the couch after they underwent the second organismic panic. Later, as he gained more experience treating such patients, he used the couch much earlier and often from the beginning.

After the second organismic panic, the fusing–disconnecting cycle, for all practical purposes, disappears and the nature of the patient's introjection and identification of the analyst image undergoes drastic modifications. Until then the patient introjects and/or identifies with "personalized" analyst images represented by a voice, smell, penis, nipple, and so on, often to quickly project them. Furthermore, during the initial phase, the act of introjection and the state of identification are accompanied by gross fantasies that can be considered cannibalistic. For example, the patient fantasizes eating the analyst, or part of the analyst enters the patient through various body orifices. After the second emotional flooding within the treatment process, the cannibalistic fantasies fade away as the patient becomes involved in more sophisticated and less "personalized" internalization acts and identification processes. The patient identifies with the analyst's ego functions.

However, observable fusing–disconnecting and internalization-externalization cycles continue to appear at times. They occur during the sessions and do not usually become generalized. Furthermore, now the patient can control these processes and this control is a good indication that their identifications with the analyst's observing functions in an atmosphere of a true therapeutic alliance is taking place, not unlike the ones that can be seen during the treatment of neurotic individuals. As Vamık Volkan reports:

> One day Jane, now being treated on the couch, reported losing the boundaries of her back while lying there (representing her fusing her body image with me or entering into my womb). She experienced high anxiety, but not an emotional flooding. The most interesting thing was that in spite of her anxiety she could "play" with her experience. Jane said that the couch had turned into a swimming pool and that she was floating above the water. She began moving her arms in order not to sink into my couch. She was also uncertain where her back ended

and where the couch began. Sitting behind her I stayed silent and let her experience this fusing, waiting to see what would develop. When the session ended, she got up and left my office without anxiety.

The next day she lost the boundaries of her back once more while lying on the couch. But this time she had come prepared. She opened her purse and pulled out a sharp pencil and stuck it into her hand. With anxiety, but also with a playful attitude, she reported that she felt pain. "But," she said, "I now know that my hand and my body belong to me." She was in control of disconnecting her self-image from my image (the couch). She was like an infant who was discovering her body boundaries and also psychologically individuating from me. In order to accomplish this, she had, in a sophisticated and silent way identified with the analyst's analyzing functions and his ability to understand her object relations conflicts.

CHAPTER 22

"Sophisticated" identifications and externalizations

In time, adults suffering from schizophrenia begin establishing "sophisticated" identifications with their analyst, using him or her as a role model (a patient, without being aware of what she is doing, takes classes to be a teacher after seeing a news item about her analyst's receiving a teaching award). Or they establish identifications with the analyst in order to strengthen or gain ego functions, which were weak or not previously available to them (after receiving a "No" response from the analyst, a patient becomes capable of using this word effectively in situations that appropriately call for it, while previously he was unable to say the word "No"). They also become capable of effectively using "sophisticated" projections in the service of belonging to their communities and large groups, such as an ethnic group.

In his books, *The Need to Have Enemies and Allies* (1988) and *Blind Trust* (2004a) Vamık Volkan illustrated that in the evolution of feelings of belonging to an ethnic, national, religious, or even ideological large group, one finds the psychology of unintegrated early self and object images. In "normal" development, a child—for practical purposes at around 36 months of life—integrates his or her "good" (libidinally contaminated) and "bad" (aggressively contaminated) self and object images (Kernberg, 1970, 1976, 1984; Mahler & Furer, 1968). But this integration is never total. Some images, associated with peak negative or positive affects, remain unintegrated. Later such unintegrated images may be subjected to repression and may appear, for example, only in dreams. Vamık Volkan noted that the assigning (externalizing) of these unintegrated images, by receiving the support and the blessing of the adults in the child's environment to *suitable targets*, is another major way the child deals with remaining unintegrated images. Otherwise, the child's—and later the adult's—integrated self and object representations will be bothered and threatened by the influence of the unintegrated images. The child—and later the adult—would be prone to having object relations conflict.

The "suitable targets" are culturally sanctioned and are therefore stable and constant reservoirs that contain the child's unintegrated "good" and "bad" images. Such reservoirs, as protosymbols (Werner & Kaplan, 1984) enhance a person's ethnic or other large-group affiliation and they also enhance the child's feelings about "enemy" groups. For example, a Finnish child "learns" to externalize his or her unintegrated "good" self and object images into the sauna, which becomes a protosymbol for the child of what it is to be a Finnish person. Only later will more complicated and sophisticated representations of other things such as the Finnish mythology, Kaleva, heroes, glories, wars won and lost, connect the Finnish child with his or her Finnishness as well as with the sauna as a symbol of being Finnish. A pig, for a Turkish child in Cyprus becomes a shared target for unintegrated "bad" self and object images and also the protosymbol of the "other," the Greek Cypriot. The pig is a stable and constant "negative" reservoir for the Cypriot Turkish child who, due to Muslim culture, will not eat (introject) the pig. The "bad" images externalized into the pig will not boomerang.

Such early, shared suitable targets are psychologically utilized to initiate the "normal" belonging to a large group as well as "normal" prejudice against the "enemy" group. Problems can arise when the early environment fails to provide feelings of belonging to a group as well as suitable targets of the externalization of the bad objects. For example, this may occur in small children of refugees or immigrants who are having serious realistic and emotional problems adjusting to a new location. Two of the symptoms of some adults with schizophrenia are directly, and at least partly, related to a failure to find suitable targets for externalization during their early childhood and an obvious absence of any large group (such as ethnic group) involvement.

The child's and his or her caretakers' psychological activities in the evolution of the child's large-group sentiments and prejudices are included in the child's mind-building "test tube." If a child is going to evolve an infantile psychotic self, these ingredients are missing or, in an opposite direction, are exaggerated. In other words, the ingredients are not "normal." In a clinical setting, when the adult psychotic self becomes the "voice" of the infantile psychotic self, we see individuals who seem to have no meaningful connection to the large groups they belong to, no sense of ethnicity, for example. And in other cases we see the opposite. In an attempt to control and "repair" the infantile psychotic self, the "envelope" absorbs an abnormal degree of large-group affiliation. The adult suffering from schizophrenia may exhibit a picture of high-level religiosity or may appear as a super-ethnic person.

After the second, therapeutic—"organismic panic," the patient's new and healthier enveloping self absorbs identifications with the analyst's cultural and other large-group sentiments. This is why many such patients of Vamık Volkan became interested in Turkish cooking and/ or Turkish music at this phase of their treatments. Later these patients would turn their attention to their own ethnic cooking and music. Sometimes they actually searched for suitable targets to absorb their externalized unintegrated self and object images. This would make their large-group sentiments stable and "normal." Below Vamık Volkan describes his unconscious response to one such patient who was looking for a positive suitable target:

> I had an urge, at first without knowing why, to hang on the wall of my office a picture clearly connected with my large-group identity. Right away my patient, who was in the third year of her psychoanalytic treatment with me, showed interest in my picture. When she asked me what geographical location this picture portrayed, I, very uncharacteristically and immediately told her that the location in the picture was from my home country, a place that I liked very much. I surprised myself for making such a disclosure before thinking what it would mean for the patient and for the analytic process. I realized that unconsciously I was trying to present a suitable target for my patient. I recalled

feeling irritated with her parents some weeks before hanging the picture when she was telling me how they did not provide her any large-group sentiments and pride. In my countertransference reaction, I guess, I wanted to be a better parent. After this incident my patient spontaneously began reading about Turks and their history. Soon she read the history about the ethnic group she belonged to, studied its art and songs, and told me how proud she was to belong to such a group.

CHAPTER 23

Permanent elimination of the infantile psychotic self?

After giving up the adult psychotic self and establishing a healthier one to replace it, some patients work hard to make the latter more and more stable. They develop the ability to repress and exhibit behavior patterns indicating the repression of their infantile psychotic selves, for example they do not remember some of their bizarre behavior patterns, which they exhibited only some years earlier. At least in theory, patients "shrink" their infantile psychotic selves. Some patients are able to consolidate their healthy envelopes nicely and it is possible to see their attempts to get rid of the core infantile psychotic self once and for all. These patients, after looking healthy for a while, would undergo another major therapeutic regression and actually return with the analyst to examine their psychotic core. This leads them to have a *third* organismic panic but this time truly under the gaze of their observing ego. Even when the observing ego is not functional during the actual emotional flooding, it returns immediately after the experience.

This third type of organismic panic is usually contained within one or two sessions and patients are able to collect themselves *before* the session is over. Through this experience patients allow their analyst *direct* contact with their infantile psychotic selves. They repair the pathogenic ingredients (the psychological ones) within the original mind- building "test tube" by mastering the "bad" affects and libidinalizing what passes through the "test tube" by the transference repetition of the original damaging infant/mother or child/mother interactions. They can then experientially understand the traumatic nature of these affects associated with such interactions and develop an ability to describe them in words and then resolve them.

A good example of this third type of organismic panic in the treatment of such patients comes from Jane's case. As we reported earlier her mother, who had lost Jane's sister when Jane was one-and-a-half years old, was depressed. Even while she was pregnant with Jane, she knew that her older daughter would not live because of a congenital anomaly. Furthermore, the depressed mother had a breast infection (confirmed by her mother during Jane's treatment) while nursing Jane. Because of the pain, she would abruptly remove her breast from infant Jane's mouth and then after a while, give her breast to the infant once more, and then remove it again. This interaction between the depressed mother and her baby was a faulty ingredient that was key to the development of Jane's infantile psychotic self. In the treatment, this poisonous mother/infant interaction was repeated, accompanied by flooding of "bad" emotions, and was then mastered. This dynamic has been recounted in great detail elsewhere (V. Volkan, 1995).

Briefly, during her emotional flooding, Jane experienced a "cosmic" event, in that her self-representation was simply an image of a mouth under a window of a huge breast-shaped cloud. Only after the experience could Jane talk to her analyst about the cloud as the mother's breast and the window as the mother's nipple. There was an omnipotent person (mother) in the cloud. During the experience Jane sensed, with accompanying indescribable "bad" feelings, that the omnipotent person's relationship with the mouth ceased abruptly, and when it ceased, the omnipotent person broke into "cosmic" laughter that "echoed" in Jane's mind, driving her "crazy." After her cosmic laughter experience, Jane simply moved on up the developmental ladder, experiencing oedipal conflicts and their resolution during the next year or so of her treatment.

It will be important for the reader to know that after her analysis finished Jane moved to another city and attended a university. She met and fell in love with a man and married him. They settled at a location far away from her previous home. Twice, at fifteen and then twenty-four years after finishing her analysis Jane visited her hometown, called her analyst, and came to visit him. This way her analyst had a chance to have a follow-up. He found that Jane was a happily married woman, a wonderful mother for her three children and active in societal organizations.

CHAPTER 24

Oedipal issues and
superego identifications

Often adults suffering from schizophrenia, even during the initial years of their treatments, exhibit stories or transference manifestations that resemble oedipal issues. These concerns, however, are not an expression of genuine oedipal processes in the transference. To pursue them during the initial work with adults suffering schizophrenia as such is a technical mistake. As indicated earlier, these patients sometimes "reach up" (Boyer, 1983) to the non-genuine oedipal issues in a defensive move to cover over genuine pre-oedipal conflicts. For example, when an adult male suffering from schizophrenia starts relating dreams in which he openly goes to bed with his mother (since his repression ability is weak, the oedipal wish appears in the open) the analyst may learn that this is a cover-up for the patient's murderous fantasies about his mother, or for his panic concerning a threat of separation from her image.

For adults suffering from schizophrenia, reaching the oedipal issues in a genuine way, as happened in Jane's case, means that they are experiencing this triangular relationship with a healthy core for the first time. The patient becomes like a "normal" child going through the oedipal phase. Therefore, the analyst helps the patient remove the obstacles and resistances to upward movement instead of interpreting the oedipal conflict as we do while analyzing individuals with high-level personality organizations.

When such patients go through the oedipal phase, the process is accompanied by further identifications with the analyst as they consolidate their superegos. In the literature these identifications are called "superego identifications." The patient reports "moral dilemmas" and resolves them. For example, the patient brings up an event in which she will make more money if she gives up her work ethic "standards." That night she dreams of the analyst (who represents a symbolic superego) who tells her not to give up her integrity and thus keep her self-esteem.

At the termination phase of their treatment patients with schizophrenia usually recall their previous fusing–disconnecting and internalization–externalization activities, some of their former delusions, and bizarre behavior patterns as if such phenomena existed in a bad dream (reflecting repression). The patient's increased ability to repress is impressive. Mourning the loss of the analyst, especially as a "new object," as described earlier, after the termination of the treatment becomes the crucial event for such patients to master in this very significant psychological process. The mourning over losing the analyst ushers in the further crystallization of sophisticated ego and superego identifications with the analyst image. This mastery becomes a defense against future breakdowns. For the analyst, the psychoanalytic treatment of such individuals is closely parallel to a parent seeing a child grow up.

Final thoughts on the psychoanalytic treatment of schizophrenia

The above sections have attempted to illustrate a theory about the genesis of adult schizophrenia and point out that adults suffering from schizophrenia are regressed because of the reappearance of an already existent, previously covered over fragile core (infantile psychotic self). This fragile core then becomes "re-enveloped" by a self that becomes the "voice" of this core. When these patients come to treatment they are "object hungry." However, initially they are not capable of knowing what is good for them to eat (introject) and how to keep what they eat. This understanding of adult schizophrenia brought to the patient's various types of internalizations of the images and functions of the analyst, leading to various identifications in the process of structurally modifying the patient's internal world.

We do not include a comprehensive report on the technique of psychoanalytic treatment of adults suffering from schizophrenia here. To include such a report would mean exploring other concepts, such as how the patient utilizes the analyst at certain times in their treatment as if the latter is a transitional object, or countertransference issues. These concepts are covered in detail elsewhere (V. Volkan, 1995).

As was previously mentioned the application of psychoanalytic treatment to adults suffering from schizophrenia (and it is important again to point out that this does not necessarily apply to those people suffering from severe chronic and/or medicated schizophrenia) has become or is becoming a "lost art", at least in the United States. While it may be a small subset of people suffering from schizophrenia who may benefit from a psychoanalytic approach to treatment, the theory described above is useful in helping to understand the dynamics of other object relations pathology, such as psychotic breaks in people suffering from borderline personality disorder or the dissociative experience of being possessed (K. Volkan, 2020b).

Also, it may be possible to adapt some of the theory described here, as well as the techniques derived from it, to help adults suffering from chronic schizophrenia, whose disease derives primarily from genetic or structural origins, and who are typically medicated. Since this group seems overrepresented in the population of people suffering from schizophrenia, the extension of the psychotherapeutic work here to this population would be especially helpful.

Part IV

Cultural elements in schizophrenia

CHAPTER 25

Schizophrenia and culture

So far, we have explicated the psychodynamics in individuals suffering from schizophrenia. This theory presented above gives rise to a number of insights related to treatment of people suffering from schizophrenia. In this Part we will examine the relationship of schizophrenia to culture and give some examples of how schizophrenia and schizophrenic-like syndromes manifest in various places around the world. Our list is by no means exhaustive. We have included examples that indicate, and in some instances explicate, some of the psychodynamic theory of schizophrenia that is outlined above. We hypothesize that while the overall category of schizophrenia as a mental illness is more or less universal, variations of schizophrenia exist that are due to pressures exerted by varying external environments and childrearing practices, as well as native beliefs about the disease.

There have been a number of studies that have focused on changes on the presentation of schizophrenic illness and variation in behavior across cultures and ethnic groups. For instance, people who have origins in the Indian subcontinent tend to present with excessive worry and irritability, while Afro-Caribbean people tend to present with delusions and paranoid ideation (Saravanan et al., 2007b). Turkish patients suffering from schizophrenia were found to exhibit more inappropriate and inane behavior than American patients suffering from the disease. The Turkish schizophrenia sufferers also displayed more euphoric behavior, while being more depersonalized, disorganized, and dissociated when compared to patients suffering from schizophrenia in America (Çetingök et al., 1990).

In his study of Irish and Italian patients suffering from schizophrenia, Marvin Opler (1959) found that the Italians were more likely to exhibit overtly homosexual behaviors, have other behavioral disorders (which we might interpret as positive symptoms), be more rejecting of authority, have less fixed delusions, have more somatic complaints, and less chronic alcoholism than their Irish counterparts. The Irish group of people suffering from schizophrenia was found to be more preoccupied with sin and guilt, less likely to have behavioral disorders, more likely to be compliant towards authorities, have more fixed delusions, have less somatic complaints, and have higher levels of chronic alcoholism than the Italian patients.

Opler concluded that it was possible to distinguish different groups among his patients with schizophrenia by their distinct cultural backgrounds and the patterns that each cultural group expressed through the stress of family conflicts. Irish families were characterized by having the mother as the central authority figure while fathers were seen as shadowy ineffectual figures in the home. The Irish male patients had been infantilized to some degree and not allowed to individuate. This resulted in anxiety and hostility being related to their mothers in most of the Irish patients. The Italians demonstrated a pattern opposite of the Irish patients, with father figures (fathers and older male siblings) being dominant in the home. This brought out expressions of hostility when there were poorly repressed conflicts with a father figure in the home. The father figures showed marked rejection of the patients, with mothers also subtly rejecting the patients and favoring the elder sons. The mothers were also neglected by the fathers and encouraged impulsiveness and hostile acting out on the part of the patients with their father figures. This resulted in the Italian patients showing emotional overflow in the form of talking too much, curious mannerisms, over-expressed grinning and laughing, and assaultiveness. They were also more likely to attempt suicide. This resulted in the Italian patients not being as paranoid as the Irish.

The Irish patients suffering from schizophrenia demonstrated more constriction of emotion, as well as a tendency to replace action with fantasy. This resulted in more delusions and paranoia. Some of the delusions took the form of persecutory thoughts related to guilt and sin as well as distortion of body image in some cases. Several of the Irish cases expressed these types of delusions by referring to a *vagina dentata*—a toothed, castrating vagina.

Another study found that individuals suffering from schizophrenia who live in developing nations are three times more likely to exhibit violent behavior than schizophrenia sufferers from developed nations. Assaultive behavior was found to be associated with positive symptoms as well as problems with alcohol abuse (Volavka et al., 1997).

CHAPTER 26

Causal beliefs related to schizophrenia

Even though presenting symptoms and behaviors may be different across cultures, the underlying schizophrenia processes can be seen as the same (Saravanan et al., 2007b). However, the attributed causes of schizophrenia can vary according to culture and exposure to Western biomedical conceptions of the disease. In one study African Americans with family members diagnosed with schizophrenia reported biological causes as the most common explanation of the disease. Personality, esoteric, and societal explanations were also important to family members of individuals suffering from schizophrenia (Mulder, 2009).

Another study compared British and Chinese beliefs about the origins, behavioral manifestations, and treatment of schizophrenia. Chinese people were found to have more religious and superstitious beliefs about the cause of schizophrenia and were more likely to frame treatment for the disease around non-scientific beliefs and traditional Chinese medicine. British people explained the causes of schizophrenia in biological, psychological, and sociological terms and framed treatment of the disease according to this view. The Chinese had more negative attitudes and beliefs about schizophrenic behavior than the British (Furnham & Wong, 2007).

These findings may be reflective of different modes of thinking that are predominant in British and Chinese cultures. While Western thought is based on an Aristotelian goal-oriented logic that is centered on the self, Chinese thought is largely based on a Confucian ideal where social relationships are seen as variations and extensions of the family dynamic. Therefore, thinking among the Chinese is more closely related to social context as well as being influenced by indigenous Daoist beliefs and practices (Varvin & Rosenbaum, 2014).

In a study in Bali, close relatives were more likely to believe in supernatural explanations as the cause of schizophrenia than natural causes. Compared with relatives who listed a natural cause as most important (14 relatives, or 36%), relatives who believed in supernatural causes of schizophrenia were generally older, had less education, and had a family member suffering from schizophrenia who had not received psychiatric treatment (Kurihara et al., 2006).

In South India 70% of patients suffering from schizophrenia in one study attributed their disease to spiritual and mystic elements, while 22% believed in a biomedical model of their illness. Patients suffering from schizophrenia who believed in a biomedical model of the disease had higher levels of insight. Being female, having a low level of education, and use of traditional healers was associated with spiritual/mystical beliefs about schizophrenia, while having a high level of insight was associated with biomedical beliefs about the illness (White et al., 2008). While some insight was inversely related to symptom severity, there was a stronger association of insight with anxiety, wanting to seek help, and perception of change. The ability to understand schizophrenic symptoms as part of a disease in self and others, as opposed to supernatural forces, was strongly associated with insight. However, this view of insight may fail to account for culturally valid explanatory frameworks for schizophrenia (Ptak & Lachmann, 2003).

In a study examining attribution of emotional reactions to schizophrenia, Mexican individuals perceived negative schizophrenic symptoms as less controllable when compared to the perceptions of Anglo-American individuals (Weisman & López, 1997).

Religious beliefs and schizophrenia

There may be a relationship between harmful religious/supernatural beliefs and schizophrenia. Bhavsar and Bhugra (2008) suggest that delusions can be generated and maintained through family expectations and religious rituals. Delusions supported by religion may also lead to harm to self or others. Certainly, religious delusions may have neurobiological origins. Studies have found that patients with post-epileptic seizure psychosis may experience hyper-religiosity. Although there are surely psychological and cultural factors at play, there is a strong likelihood of a neurological involvement. This involvement may include the limbic system and the neocortex. It may be that the so-called "ecstatic" religious experience is related to changes in the frontal and temporal regions of the right hemisphere of the brain (Devinsky & Lai, 2008).

Effects of schizophrenia across cultures

In addition to beliefs about the causes and how to treat schizophrenia, rates of marriage and fertility of people suffering from schizophrenia may differ by culture. As might be expected individuals suffering from schizophrenia are less likely to marry and have children than non-sufferers. It is not known, however, whether this is due to the effects of the illness itself or the impaired social cognition or social milieu among people suffering from schizophrenia.

One study compared marriage, relationship stability, and fertility rates of white British, Caribbean, and Asian subjects suffering from schizophrenia. It was found that British and Caribbean subjects (but not Asians) had decreased rates of stable relationships, marriage, fertility, and number of children compared to normal controls. These findings suggest a decrease in marriage and sexual behavior are associated with schizophrenia, but that this is influenced by society and culture (Hutchinson et al., 1999).

Immigration and schizophrenia

There is an immense body of literature and a long history of research linking schizophrenia to immigration. Ørnulv Ødegård (1932) was one of the first to study mental illness among immigrants. He hypothesized that Norwegian immigrants to the United States had poor social adaptation before they immigrated and were essentially "weak" and predisposed to mental illness. In other words, there was a selection bias, whereby people predisposed to insanity were more likely to immigrate than the general population.

It is likely that individuals suffering from schizophrenia who are immigrants may have a different cultural background that the professionals who provide their treatment (Fearon et al., 2006; Gibson et al., 2013; Leão et al., 2006; Simpson, 1995). Therefore, it is important to treat schizophrenia among immigrants in ways that mobilize cultural explanations. There are many case studies in the literature that provide positive examples of this way of working with patients suffering from schizophrenia (W.-C. Hwang, 2007; Kastrup et al., 2008; Mausbach et al., 2008; Saravanan et al., 2007a).

Individuals who migrate from developing countries to England and the Netherlands are known to have high rates of schizophrenia. Also, among non-white, non-immigrants, the incidence of schizophrenia goes up as when their ethnic presence is reduced in the place where they live. One explanation put forward to explain this phenomenon is "social defeat." This term is derived from ethological studies where one animal physically defeats another animal. The defeated animal must then constantly display submissive behavior. This type of defeat and submissive behavior has been shown in rats to increase dopaminergic activity in the meso-limbic system that is thought to be associated with schizophrenia. Isolation increases this effect while removal from the physically dominating animal reduces it.

The idea that this sort of dynamic could increase schizophrenia rates among non-white people who find themselves living in a white-dominant society is quite plausible (Luhrmann, 2007). Looked at from another view, sociocentric indicators that were related to ethnic culture were found to mediate differences in symptoms in Latino and Black schizophrenia sufferers, compared to white patients suffering from the disease. These sociocentric indicators were found to reduce symptoms for non-white patients suffering from schizophrenia in the study. This may demonstrate that people suffering from schizophrenia who have strong cultural support may have reduced symptoms of the disorder (Brekke & Barrio, 1997).

CHAPTER 27

Object relations and culture

It is known that the presentation and interpretation of schizophrenia, including its associated behavior and symptoms, can differ across cultures. However, object relations pathology has been demonstrated in populations of people suffering from schizophrenia when measured across cultures. One example is a study by Morris Bell and Wilze Bruscato (2002), who studied normal populations and populations of people suffering from schizophrenia in Brazil and the United States. They found that people in their sample suffering from schizophrenia had object relations deficits regardless of country.

Object relations theory centers on how people and things in the external world form mental representations, beginning in infancy, in the human mind. It also includes the nature of the relationships between mental representations and the external world. Motivated by drives, object representations emerge through the interaction between infants and their primary caregiver, which in Western societies is usually the mother. These form enduring patterns of relationship leading to feelings of security when the primary caregiver is absent, which in turn, during normal development, results in stable psychic structures and a healthy sense of self. In general, this pattern of normal development is seen in humans everywhere. However, since the objects that are internalized as mental representations can differ from culture to culture it would stand that object representations and their pattern of relationships may show some differences across cultures. As Jeffrey Applegate (1990) says, "The ways in which these internal representations become expressed in behavior will vary according to both actual environmental surroundings and their internal representations" (p. 88).

The culture surrounding infants and the actual environment in which they live will be reflected in their internal mental environment. This can occur in a number of ways, most prominently through play in what Donald Winnicott (1971) labeled "potential space" that is the infant's emerging awareness of separation between self and others. As he says, "In order to give a place to playing, I postulated a potential space between the baby and mother. This potential space varies a very great deal according to the life experiences of the baby in relation to the mother or mother-figure" (p. 41).

Separation–individuation experiences aided by transitional phenomena emerge in the potential space and are crucial for normal development. However, the details of how infants experience the potential space and develop specific patterns of object relations can be influenced by culturally mediated elements. There are three areas where cultural variations can play a role in infants' developing object representations and sense of self: family structure, child rearing practices, and experience of ethnicity or race. We will explore these ideas briefly below drawing primarily from Jeffrey Applegate's (1990) work.

In the developed Western countries early development has been viewed through the lens of a dyadic relationship between infant and mother. In this family structure the role of fathers, siblings, grand-parents, etc. has been minimized, at least in early infancy. Yet, Applegate (1990) citing Robert Emde (1981) and Daniel Stern (1985) reports that even newborn infants are able to discriminate and interact with a wide variety of people. More recent research has demonstrated that even before one year of age infants are not only aware of others but are increasingly able to make causal inferences about how these others manipulate the environment and communicate with each other (Kosugi & Fujita, 2001).

In other words, babies are capable of developing relationships with multiple objects, and presumably internalizing mental representations of these objects as well. This object relations plurality is often seen in other cultures (F. Lieberman, 1984). This may arise because families are defined differently across cultures. For instance, a family structure may have multiple primary caregivers who can gratify an infant's dependency needs and serve as additional protection against feelings of anxiety when compared to the dyadic mother–child relationship that is common in the Western developed world. This in turn affects the infant's exploration of the potential space, resulting in less need for transitional objects for self-soothing and perhaps more broadly defined culturally mediated transitional phenomena.

Child rearing practices and beliefs vary widely across cultures though the idea that helpless infants are dependent on adults and need protection seems to be universal. The ways in which infants are taken care of and protected varies greatly across cultures and is related to beliefs about birth, identity, and weaning. These beliefs can influence the developing child's object relations patterns in a number of ways. In the Western developed world birth is generally a medically mediated process that happens in a hospital or hospital-like setting. This tends to make birth in the Western developed world an isolating event. Typically, no or few family members are present during the birth event, and the baby is taken from the mother, inoculated, tested, and if deemed necessary, given treatment for various things.

While there has been a movement in some developed countries to have birthing centers that encourage family involvement and the bonding of the mother and baby after the birth, these are not universal. In contrast, in most other places, giving birth is seen as a natural event, occurring most often in the home, attended by a midwife with the help of the father and wife's mother. Most importantly, the mother, but also the father and other family members (such as grandparents and aunts and uncles) immediately begin to bond with the baby. This type of non-medicalized birth experience may also elicit strong feelings of attachment in parents and family members and presumably eases the baby's frightening transition into the outside world. It seems likely that this could have some impact in the child's object relations development. Likewise, the presence of multiple primary caregivers can affect child rearing practices such as weaning, feeding, and soothing.

Cultures differ in the timing of these three areas of child rearing, as well as the motivation of behavior related to each. In some cultures, weaning may not occur for years and may happen gradually according to the child's interest in other types of nourishment. Conversely, in other cultures weaning may be abrupt and decided according to the mother's needs. Feeding an infant can be an occasion of emotional attachment (which is classically related to breastfeeding) or just the provision of nourishment. Feelings generated around feeding can be centered on a sole mother figure or a group of primary caregivers (grandmother, neighbors, wet nurse, etc.). Likewise, for soothing of infants, where in some cultures they may be left on their own for hours at a time and others where they are picked up and held the minute they cry.

At a somewhat later age the way in which the child begins to identify with their ethnicity or race and becomes aware of how their ethnicity or race is perceived in the world around them can affect their internal object world. This in turn can affect the child's separation–individuation. Ethnic and racial characteristics such as skin color or language can influence the potential space. Ethnic intergenerational trauma can also be transmitted to the child (V. Volkan, 1988). When this occurs, the child identifies with past group trauma and unconsciously plays out ethnic conflict in their own psychic makeup, continuing its perpetration into the future. As Vamık Volkan (2004b) writes:

> Clinical investigations of members of groups that have suffered a massive trauma at the hands of an enemy group reveal that although each individual has his or her own unique identity and personal reaction to the trauma, all (or almost all) group members have developed injured self-images as a result. Studies of the second and third generations of a group that has suffered such a trauma (such as the children and grandchildren of Holocaust survivors) clearly show that the mental representation of the shared tragedy is transmitted to subsequent generations in varying levels of intensity. (p. 48)

It should be clear from the above section on the object relations dynamics in the schizophrenic personality how the cultural influence on object relations patterns could affect the development of a schizophrenic self-structure or cause someone with a schizophrenic self-structure to experience organismal panic and descend into schizophrenia. Likewise, it is possible to speculate that some cultural influences on object relations could protect a child from developing schizophrenia.

For instance, having a family structure that includes multiple primary caregivers might be protective against the development of schizophrenia. Multiple primary caregivers could provide more libidinally toned object representations that could lead to better object integration and less hostile unintegrated object representations. This could compensate for genetic or structural predispositions to schizophrenia, making the infant more resilient. On the other hand, as Vamık Volkan (2019) describes, if there is intense conflict between multiple primary caregivers this situation may make the child's developing his or her integration function difficult. Also, child rearing practices such as abrupt weaning or ignoring the child's need for soothing could have a negative effect.

Ethnic and/or racial identification as well as transgenerational trauma may promote schizophrenia (M. J. Miller, 2011). The idea that object relations and object relations pathology related to schizophrenia can vary tremendously across cultures can be seen in the examples given in the next chapter. This is supported by the research on schizophrenia and immigration we presented above.

CHAPTER 28

Culture-bound schizophrenia

There are several syndromes that appear related to schizophrenia and its variants found among the cultures of the world. Marvin Opler (1959) says, "... schizophrenias are not a collection of air-tight entities, since different cultural backgrounds defined variations in family and social structure, reflecting into pathology. As such schizophrenias could highlight, rather than obscure, severely emotionalized conflicts rooted in culture" (pp. 430–431). Some examples of culture related schizophrenic-like syndromes are presented below. This list is by no means exhaustive but should illuminate both some differences and similarities in the presentation of schizophrenic-like illnesses found across cultures worldwide.

In addition to looking at expressions of schizophrenic illness by different cultural groups, it is possible to also look at distinct related syndromes that have arisen in various cultures. Four culture-bound disorders are presented as brief but specific examples of how culturally related syndromes linked to psychosis can be expressed in different cultures. These examples, *wendigo* psychosis, *qigong* psychosis, *amafufunyana*, and *Saora* disorder share many similarities in symptoms, but differ in how they develop, initially present, and resolve.

Wendigo psychosis

Let us start with a quote from woodsman, adventurer, and storyteller Bob Cary:

> "What are you doing Bob?" I turned to meet the stolid mahogany visage of Native American wilderness guide Stanley Owl, who was portaging canoes and gear for a group of fishermen.
>
> "We're shooting a movie," I said. "I see that." Stan's dark eyes flickered over the scene. "But what are YOU doing?" "Uh … well … ." I realized that Stanley would not approve my venture. "I'm going to take the canoe by myself up around the base of the falls so I'll kind of be silhouetted against the foam … then take the main current and shoot the rapids past the camera."
>
> "Can't do that," Stanley stated evenly.
>
> "What do you mean I can't?"
>
> "There's a wendigo in those rapids," Stanley replied without a flicker of emotion.
>
> "Wendigo? Ah, come on, Stan, that's a lot of old Indian superstition … you don't believe in that stuff, do you?"
>
> Stan's eyes flickered a trifle. "Five years ago a Forest Service ranger and I tried to run it. The canoe got torn apart and we both got smashed up pretty bad. He was in the hospital for three weeks."
>
> "That wasn't any wendigo, you guys just screwed up."
>
> "No …" Stan said softly. "There's something in there. You can't make it Bob." (1996, pp. 111–112)

In the story above Bob indeed tries to run the rapids and has a strange mishap that destroys his boat and threatens his life. He takes the existence of the wendigo more seriously afterwards. What is this supposed wendigo creature?

Wendigo psychosis (sometimes transliterated as *windigo, weetego, widigo*, etc.) is a culture-bound syndrome found among Algonquin speaking Native Americans that include the Cree, Innu, Naskapi, Ojibwe, and Saulteaux peoples. Wendigo supposedly means "the evil one that devours" in the Cree language. The wendigo psychosis is the so-called delusional belief that one will turn into an evil cannibalistic monster or evil spirit.

This can be accompanied by schizophrenic-like negative or positive symptoms including paranoia. There are also cultural beliefs about the wendigo that support the syndrome in individuals. The wendigo is a creature that was once a man. But because he is starving in an isolated winter environment, the man begins to crave human flesh, eventually succumbing to his cannibalistic desires, turning into a monster or an unseen evil spirit. The monster or spirit is a malevolent man-eater who also acts with hostility towards those it encounters. Later, after the incursion of the white man, the wendigo is also seen as a nature spirit who keeps nature in balance, taking vengeance against those who disturb this balance. This meaning is clear in this account (Lindberg, 1974):

> But when Pop asked again about the varmints pressing in from the hills the way they did, then John said something about the spirit of the season. What's that? snaps Pop, not believing he heard right. Wendigo. That's our name for him, says John. And who might that be? When the year runs as it always does, then Wendigo stays asleep, because he knows we do not need him. But when the weather turns bad, and the rains dry up, and a hard winter is coming, then Wendigo comes close to us to help us in our need. Is that what you were doing in the woods for three days, praying for help from a heathen woods devil? John looked at Pop in something of the way that he looked at Brady's rifle when Brady threw him off his land. Then he looked far off at the woods and spoke in a flat voice: We do not pray to beg. We make ourselves clean and open to the spirit. We go a long way alone, and we do not eat or drink or sleep. We make a gift of ourselves because Wendigo keeps the good seasons from us only when we have done wrong. (p. 9)

This story ends with the bad guy, Brady, being attacked by the wendigo and spirited away never to be seen again, and in all likelihood eaten by the monster.

There has been some speculation that the wendigo (as well as other cryptids, such as the *Toonijuks* of the Eskimos, the Alaskan *Devils* of Thomas Bay, and the *Sasquatch* of British Columbia), may be remnants of sub-hominid populations that lived on the American continent before proto-Native American people migrated across the Bering Strait (Sanderson, 1963).

People supposedly begin to suffer from the delusion that they will become a wendigo during periods of starvation. One of the theories about the disorder was that it was due to either lack of fat in the diet or a deficiency in some vitamin or enzyme (Rohrl, 1970). This theory has for the most part been debunked since other people living in similar conditions and subject to restricted caloric intake during the winter months do not report turning into cannibalistic monsters. In a much older case history immoderate singing and dancing was thought to protect against becoming a wendigo (McGee, 1972). It is possible that that some institutionalized cannibalism existed among the Algonquin people. Two main forms of cannibalism are endo- and exo-cannibalism. Endo-cannibalism is where a group of people consume people within their group, typically as part of a funeral ritual. Exo-cannibalism is where a group consumes people outside their group, usually in the context of aggression in order to gain the power of an enemy or as an insult.

For the Algonquin people the wendigo myth provides some framework for the act of endo-cannibalism when exo-cannibalism is not possible. Harold McGee (1972) offers us this explanation though it concerns Native people somewhat to the east of the Algonquins:

> During the period when the windigo is most active people are dispersed in small extended family or nuclear family camps. Who would be eaten if there existed a choice between a kinsman and non-kinsman? One harsh winter the Micmac near Miscou consumed a Basque boy left among them to learn their language … Although I have not examined all cases of early cannibalism for the sub-arctic it would appear likely that the victim was chosen on the basis of whose relatives offered the least threat and who offered the most meat. (p. 245)

Given that disorders such as *Piblokto* have been shown to be caused by over consumption of vitamin A among the Inuit, nutritional causes of wendigo may deserve further study using more modern nutritional assessment methodology (Landy, 1985).

Wendigo psychosis has also been related to severe anxiety neurosis centered upon food among the Ojibwa people. This manifests as delusions, paranoia, depression, violent behavior, and obsession with cannibalism that are the hallmarks of wendigo psychosis (Landes, 1938). Some doctors treating wendigo psychosis make the case for it being a conversion syndrome (Hagen & Schokking, 1990).

One startling case of wendigo psychosis gives some psychological insight into the psychodynamics of the disorder (Hallowell, 1936):

> One morning a young man of about 20 years of age on getting up, said he felt a strong inclination to eat his sister; as he was a steady young man, and a promising hunter, no notice was taken of this expression; the next morning he said the same and repeated the same several times in the day for a few days. His parents attempted to reason him out of this horrid inclination; he was silent and gave them no answer; his sister and her husband became alarmed, left the place and went to another camp. He became aware of it and then said he must have human flesh to eat, and would have it; in other respects, his behavior was cool, calm and quiet. His father and relations were much grieved; argument had no effect on him, and he made them no answer to their questions. The camp became alarmed, for it was doubtful who would be his victim. His father called the men to a council, where the state of the young man was discussed, and their decision was, that an evil spirit had entered into him, and was in full possession of him to make him become a Man Eater (a Weetego). The father was found fault with for not having called to his assistance a Medicine Man, who by sweating and his songs to the tambour and rattle might have driven away the evil spirit, before it was too late. Sentence of death was passed on him, which was to be done by his father. The young man was called ... [and] ... informed of the resolution taken, to which he said, "I am willing to die"; the unhappy father arose, and placing a cord about his neck strangled him, to which he was quite passive; after about two hours, the body was carried to a large fire, and burned to ashes, not the least bit of bone remaining. This was carefully done to prevent his soul and evil spirit which possessed him from returning to this world and appearing at his grave; as they believe the souls of those who are buried can, and may do, as having a claim to the bones of their bodies. It may be thought that the council acted a cruel part in ordering the father to put his son to death, when they could have ordered it by the hands of another person. This was

done, to prevent the law of retaliation; which had it been done by the hands of another person, might have been made a pretext of revenge by those who were not the friends of the person who put him to death. Such is the state of society where there are no positive laws to direct mankind. (p. 38)

This remarkable case of wendigo psychosis presents a number of psychological mechanisms at work. The young man at the center of the story shows evidence of negative symptoms of schizophrenia as well as a persistent delusion. Surprisingly, within his delusion is an obvious oedipal conflict, the "reaching up" we described earlier. The young man wants to eat his sister. It is fairly easy to read a sexual intent and, indeed inuendo, into this desire. The sister is already married and presumably older and a mother-figure to the young man. The father has to step in to prevent the eating of the sister and is obliged to strangle the young man—an act of killing reminiscent of castration.

Qigong psychosis

While the DSM-V (American Psychiatric Association, 2013) does not mention qigong psychosis, the previous version (DSM-IV) did, though not in conjunction with schizophrenic illness (American Psychiatric Association, 2000). Qigong psychosis can be used to identify psychoses related to the traditional Chinese practice of qigong exercises or to other meditation practices found mostly in the Far East (W.-C. Hwang, 2007).

Qigong is generally a type of exercise where body movements are coordinated with specific breathing patterns, visualization, or imagined feelings inside the body. There are many hundreds of different qigong exercises that make it hard to generalize about this practice. For the most part, qigong practice is done to prevent illness, to treat illness, and as a spiritual practice. Each of these different kinds of qigong has separate kinds of practices, though some do overlap. Qigong works by balancing, promoting, and maintaining the flow of Qi in the body. Qi, which is key to understanding the traditional conception of the body in China, is a type of universal energy that flows not only through the body but also throughout the world. The body is seen as a microcosm of the macrocosmic universe. The body becomes diseased when the Qi in the body becomes unbalanced (deficient or in excess), or flows improperly (stagnant or out of control). Qigong practice aims to correct these types of imbalance (Y. Lee & Hu, 1993). Medical and psychological research is now providing evidence of the healthfulness of qigong practice (Guadalupe et al., 2017; Hiraoka et al., 1997; Y. Lee & Hu, 1993).

Since mind and Qi are intimately related, qigong practice can also enhance mental clarity and perception and like other forms of meditation is useful for spiritual pursuits. However, this close relationship with the mind also means that certain types of qigong, if practiced improperly or by the wrong person, can adversely affect the mind. While qigong practice can possibly contribute to psychosis (Hwang, 2007), the cultural understanding of the psychotic experience itself is related to conceptions of the body and its inherent energy seen in traditional Chinese medicine.

Interestingly enough, traditionally, severe mental illness has been identified for at least 1,000 years as a possible negative side effect of improper qigong practice. For some interesting descriptions of qigong induced psychiatric symptoms see Bruce Frantzis (1993). Especially fascinating are the dangers of "Crane" style vibrating qigong practices. It is interesting to note that many of the techniques for generating power found in traditional Okinawan Karate may be related to this type of Crane qigong practice (Sells, 2000).

Russell Lim and Keh-Ming Lin (1996) present an example of qigong psychosis in the case of a fifty-seven-year-old married Chinese American male qigong practitioner. After practicing qigong for three weeks, he began to hear voices commanding him to perform qigong movements in a certain way. The patient was certain that these voices emanated from beings in another dimension. He was diagnosed with schizophreniform disorder and was treated with a neuroleptic drug that improved his symptoms. The authors were not able to conclude whether the abatement of the patient's symptoms was due to the medication or the cessation of qigong practice.

In a similar vein, Harold Kuijpers et al. (2007) describes a case of meditation-induced acute polymorphic psychosis. He concludes that meditation can be a stressor that triggers a brief reactive psychosis. Beng-Yeong Ng (1999), in a review of qigong-induced mental disorders, also concludes that such psychotic episodes are culture-bound but that the cultural elements serve as a stressor than can trigger the psychotic break in vulnerable people.

Amafufunyana

Dana Neihaus and colleagues (2004) cite two syndromes, *amafufunyana* (possession by evil spirits) and the related *ukuthwasa* (coming out or gradually appearing) that occur in a number of tribes such as the Xhosa and Zulu, in South Africa as examples of culture-bound syndromes that are used to explain psychotic or schizophrenic behavior and symptoms. Ukuthwasa often pertains to the reported appearance of ancestral spirits related to a specific clan. In this instance the experience of the syndrome can be part of the training and initiation of a novice healer (Tropp, 2003).

Amafufunyana is a syndrome where people believe they have been possessed by evil spirits (usually more than one). This possession is brought about by malicious enchantment, where a witch finds ants that have been living in a graveyard, and by association, feeding on dead people. These ants are collected and mixed up into a poisonous *idliso* or *muthi*, which is some type of substance that victims ingest or come into contact with, usually through walking over it or having it blown into their face. In fact, the act of blowing into the palm is commonly used to indicate that someone is a witch. In some cases, even dreaming about ingesting the substance is enough to cause the disorder (Ashforth, 2005).

After the victim has been exposed to the idliso they begin to experience the symptoms of the syndrome. These include hearing voices, often from the stomach and in a different language than one's own, agitation, fatigue, loss of appetite, impulsive anger and aggression, difficulty sleeping, nightmares, and suicidal behavior. The voices can become commanding, threatening, or persecutory, and at times take on the character of someone else, presumably one of the evil spirits posing as the victim. Like some kinds of psychoses amafufunyana can manifest en masse.

One case documented by Steve Edwards (1984) described 400 children who purportedly suffered from amafufunyana over a two-year period. The children exhibited painful, swollen bellies, ran out of control, rolled their eyes, and lashed out wildly. One teacher reported that if the children's bellies were squeezed, voices claiming to be the possessing spirits could be heard speaking in Zulu. In terms of Western psychology amafufunyana seems very much like a form of psychosis, but also includes elements of somatic, dissociative, and impulse control pathologies (Spanos & Gottlieb, 1979).

For the Xhosa and Zulu people these syndromes provide an emic account that gives meaning to the disorder in a way that is understood by the person who is suffering (Ensink & Robertson, 1996). Although sufferers may contextualize the syndrome according to cultural beliefs this does not prevent them necessarily from obtaining relief through Western biomedical approaches to treatment (Allen et al., 2004). In addition, the traditional cultural belief system was able to consistently differentiate between psychotic and non-psychotic syndromes (Edwards, 1984). For example, in tribes in the northern part of South Africa faith healers make a distinction between madness (*bogafi*) and amafufunyana. In fact, the treatment of mental illness (which encompasses both bogafi and amafufunyana) is one of the largest specialties practiced by faith healers in the Northern Provinces (Peltzer, 1999).

At the turn of the century faith healers (and in some instances the Christian Church) tended to see phenomena like amafufunyana as having supernatural causes while Western psychology and sociology did not. A good example of this was a case of mass amafufunyana at an Anglican school where both the traditional healers and the Church placed the blame for the epidemic on possession by evil spirits. However, a Western authority blamed the outbreak on rapid social changes leading to extreme stress and characterized the epidemic as a case of mass hysteria (Parle, 2003). A more recent study found that even with different theoretical orientations, traditional healers and modern psychologists agreed both in diagnosis and treatment modalities given limited options. Patients found both traditional healers and modern psychology about equally as helpful (Carré et al., 2011).

Saora disorder

This is a disorder that occurs among young people (teenagers to young adults) of the Saora (sometimes spelled Sora) tribe in the Andhra State along the southeast coast of India. Some Saora people also live in the hill country of Jharkhand and in Maharashtra and Madhya Pradesh. This disorder has a number of features similar to schizo-phrenia such as crying and laughing at inappropriate times, loss of memory, and a delusional belief in the presence of supernatural beings who communicate with them. The disorder has other features such as passing out and the sensation of being bitten by ants in the absence of any insects. The Saora people explain the disorder as being caused by supernatural spirit beings or gods. It is believed that these gods choose young people for a sort of spiritual wedding. This wedding in no way prevents or invalidates romantic relationships and marriage with other human beings, but instead entails the person and god being connected throughout life. If a young person refuses to marry a god, or there is some disagreement among the gods over who should marry whom, the supernatural beings then cause the symptoms. If the young person marries a god, then the symptoms will cease. It is thought that young people who have gone through the disorder have some ability to be sensitive to the spirit world and therefore will make good shamans. The local village shaman will take those who come through the disorder as apprentices, training them to heal people by intervening with the supernatural forces. Among the Saora becoming a shaman bestows status and respect upon the young person so chosen for this profession (Krippner, 2019).

It should be noted that the Saora have their own gods that may or may not be related to the larger Hindu culture in which the Saora exist. It is thought that the Saora were once a dominant tribe in southern India that possessed a complicated culture. However, over the ages they have become diminished compared to their past and consist mostly of farmers (Elwin, 1955). There has been a push by Hindu nationalists to convert the Saora to Hinduism that has caused considerable conflict. Some Saora have also been converted to Christianity (Vitebsky, 1993, 2017).

It is possible that the young people afflicted with the disorder are experiencing a psychotic break that may be triggered by societal stressors and conditions. The Saora are mainly poor subsistence farmers and young people born into this society have little chance of a life other than what their parents have. This may be worse if the young person is a woman since the Saora tend towards polygamy and are endogamous, marrying within the tribe. A young woman may be married to a man who has multiple wives, which could further constrain her position in the family. Symptoms of Saora disorder may be related to the rather bleak outlook that is the fate of most Saoras in their teens and early twenties. They might want to leave the village, seek out an education, move to a big city for employment, and not live their lives as subsistence farmers, but are under intense psychological and social pressure not to do these things. The symptoms of the disorder may serve as a sort of pressure relief valve and a way out of the fate that awaits them. Resolution of the sickness often results in a change of career path, that is, becoming a shaman, which we can assume is preferable to subsistence farming. Interestingly, a similar sort of dynamic was found among ultraorthodox Jewish patients who experienced a psychotic break within a month of marriage (Fisch, 1992).

CHAPTER 29

Psychoanalysis and syndromes of culture-bound schizophrenia

What we described in the previous chapter are just a few examples from around the world and many more could have been included. Disorders like *Koro* (Ramamourty et al., 2014), *Dhat* (Udina et al., 2013), *Susto* (Consoli et al., 2013), *Abidjan-Niger Psychosis* (Verlingue, 1986), *Ataque* and *Nervios* (Lewis-Fernáandez, 1996), *Phii Pob* (Suwanlert, 1976), etc., have been related to psychosis. Some of these other disorders are clearly variants of psychosis while we can be less sure of others. Given lack of diagnostic precision and uncertainty it becomes easy to attribute many different culturally related syndromes and phenomena to some sort of variation of schizophrenia. An example might be found in *Phii Pob*, which occurs in Thailand; it is a form of spirit possession in which a person is inhabited by a spirit, but the spirit can also possess others nearby. This form of delusion has some similarities to Capgras syndrome where the sufferer believes that people close to them have been taken over by imposters (Berson, 1983; K. Volkan, 2020a).

Conversely, we also see attribution of known forms of psychosis to some sort of cultural uniqueness. An instance of the latter can perhaps be found with *Abidjan-Niger* psychosis, which occurs among migrant workers in what is now Burkina Faso. This disorder has been described as an acute polymorphic psychotic disorder. It is thought to occur among individuals who have anal compulsive character organization (Verlingue, 1986). While there were some cultural elements to the delusions, which were chiefly persecutory, the disorder presents much like brief reactive psychosis and resolves quickly with medication. *Susto*, *Ataque*, and *Nervios* are likely cultural variants of acute and post-traumatic disorders as well as anxiety disorders rather than schizophrenia. Koro and Dhat have more in common with body dysmorphic disorder than with schizophrenia even though they have strong delusional symptomology.

The culture-bound forms of psychosis described here could also be seen as overlapping with other disorders. However, they present a number of etiological factors that seem to cross cultural boundaries. Oedipal distortion in the family can be seen among the Irish, Italian, and Ojibwa versions of psychosis. This can be seen as instances of "reaching up," which we described earlier. Clearly early family dynamics play a role in determining the specific symptoms and traits of the psychosis.

Italian patients suffering from schizophrenia and wendigo sufferers appear to express more hostility. For the Irish and the Saora, religious and cultural restraint in the sufferers appears to play an important role. The Xhosa, Zulu, Ojibwa, and Saora include an element of spirit possession that adds a flavor of dissociation to their forms of psychosis. Qigong psychosis may have more in common with *Abidjan-Niger* psychosis where a stressor can trigger a psychotic reaction.

Last words

The research and writing on schizophrenia are vast, extending over a wide area of different spheres of medicine and psychology. In this book we reflected this truth. However, our aim has been to highlight the main points of knowledge about what is known to help us focus in on what may be beneficial for future studies. We can think of each Part of the book like a circle in a Venn diagram, with many overlapping areas that hopefully will provide future insights into schizophrenia.

In this schematic, the shaded area indicates the intersection of all areas of inquiry into schizophrenia and suggests possibilities for the future. As such, we can speculate on what this might represent.

First off, it is likely that in the future multimodal treatment for schizophrenia will be available. This will include mainstream, psycho-therapeutic, and cultural elements. There is room for improvement in each element. Mainstream understanding of the neuropathology will almost certainly become more detailed and nuanced. This is turn should lead to more targeted pharmacological treatment with fewer side effects.

Treatments based on immunity modulation, neuromodulation, and psychosurgery show much promise and may become viable options

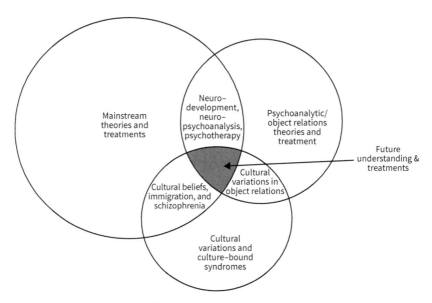

Figure 4 Intersection of inquiry into schizophrenia.

for some of those suffering from schizophrenia. Efforts to prevent schizophrenia may also be more successful. All these mainstream modalities for understanding and treating schizophrenia will be enhanced by psychoanalytic object relations theory. An understanding of the physical development of the brain will be enhanced by knowledge of the development of psychological structures. Increased correlation between structures arising in the growing brain and the phenomenology of mental structures will allow newer treatments to more precisely target schizophrenic pathology. Combination treatments could include psychoanalytic-based psychotherapy used in conjunction with improved psychopharmacology as well as with modalities like neuromodulation.

From the above examples of schizophrenia-like culture-bound disorders it can be seen that in creating newer approaches to schizophrenia it will be important for both clinicians and researchers to understand how the disorder manifests in different cultures. This approach argues against a "one size fits all" approach to understanding and possibly treating psychotic variation around the world. Understanding of religious beliefs, indigenous treatments, local medical and healing practices, as well as culturally determined family structures and external social stressors on specific cultural groups should become part of the training of mental health professionals, who are increasingly treating patients in an ever-shrinking world.

This book was written during the COVID pandemic that began in March of 2020. As we mentioned in the beginning of the book, coronaviruses can have an effect on the nervous system and the brain that can lead to an increase in cases of schizophrenia. There is no reason to believe that the SARS-2 virus will not have the same effect. Already we are hearing of neurological effects of the virus among the populations of the world.

In addition, the fear and anxiety created by the pandemic, the need for social distancing, and increased utilization of virtual relationships have and will influence human psychology. Changes in child rearing and parenting, social development, education, loss and upheaval in work, not to mention increased rates of depression and anxiety are all now a "new" reality. How these changes will affect rates of schizophrenia is unknown and, we are sure, will be studied in due time. However, the prognosis is not good.

Our hope is that this book can provide not only an overview of schizophrenia but also perhaps new ways of approaching this debilitating disorder, including news ways to conceptualize and expand treatment beyond the current paradigm, as well as new lines of research into integrative treatments that can be made available to all who need it. These different approaches are needed now and will likely be even more important in the near future.

References

Abse, D. W., & Ewing, J. A. (1960). Some problems in psychotherapy with schizophrenic patients. *American Journal of Psychotherapy, 14*: 505–519.

Adam, M. A., & Harwell, C. C. (2020). Epigenetic regulation of cortical neurogenesis; orchestrating fate switches at the right time and place. *Current Opinion in Neurobiology, 63*: 146–153.

Adams, D. D., Knight, J. G., & Ebringer, A. (2012). The autoimmune model of schizophrenia. *ISRN Psychiatry*: 758072.

Agarwal, V., Abhijnhan, A., & Raviraj, P. (2007). Ayurvedic medicine for schizophrenia. *Cochrane Database of Systematic Reviews, 4*: CD006867.

Agbeli, M. O. (2020). *Reducing Antipsychotic Medication Use in Long-term Care Settings*. Ann Arbor, MI: ProQuest Information & Learning.

Alanen, Y. O. (1993). *Skitsofrenia- syyt ja tarpeenmukainen hoito*. Helsinki: WSOY.

Albert, N., Randers, L., Allott, K., Jensen, H. D., Melau, M., Hjorthøj, C., & Nordentoft, M. (2019). Cognitive functioning following discontinuation of antipsychotic medication. A naturalistic sub-group analysis from the OPUS II trial. *Psychological Medicine, 49*: 1138–1147.

Allen, M., Naka, K., & Ishizu, H. (2004). Attacked by the gods or by mental illness? Hybridizing mental and spiritual health in Okinawa. *Mental Health, Religion & Culture, 7*: 83–107.

Alvarez-Jimenez, M., Priede, A., Hetrick, S. E., Bendall, S., Killackey, E., Parker, A. G., McGorry, P. D., & Gleeson, J. F. (2012). Risk factors for relapse following treatment for first episode psychosis: A systematic review and meta-analysis of longitudinal studies. *Schizophrenia Research, 139*: 116–128.

American Psychiatric Association (2000). *Diagnostic and Statistical Manual of Mental Disorders, 4th Edition*. Washington, DC: American Psychiatric Association.

American Psychiatric Association (2013). *Diagnostic and Statistical Manual of Mental Disorders, 5th Edition*. Washington, DC: American Psychiatric Association.

Angyal, A. (1950). The psychodynamic process of illness and recovery in a case of catatonic schizophrenia. *Psychiatry: Journal for the Study of Interpersonal Processes, 13*: 149–165.

Applegate, J. S. (1990). Theory, culture, and behavior: Object relations in context. *Child and Adolescent Social Work Journal, 7*: 85–100.

Apprey, M. (1997). The intersubjective constitution of the sense of disappearing in schizophrenia: A phenomenological description of a healthy sibling's intuitions. In: V. Volkan & S. Akhtar (Eds.), *The Seed of Madness: Constitution, Environment, and Fantasy in the Organization of the Psychotic Core* (pp. 81–109). Madison, CT: International Universities Press.

Arlow, J. A., & Brenner, C. (1964). *Psychoanalytic Concepts and the Structural Theory*. Madison, CT: International Universities Press.

Arnaiz, A., Zumárraga, M., Díez-Altuna, I., Uriarte, J. J., Moro, J., & Pérez-Ansorena, M. A. (2011). Oral health and the symptoms of schizophrenia. *Psychiatry Research, 188*: 24–28.

Ashcroft, K., Kingdon, D. G., & Chadwick, P. (2012). Persecutory delusions and childhood emotional abuse in people with a diagnosis of schizophrenia. *Psychosis: Psychological, Social and Integrative Approaches, 4*: 168–171.

Ashforth, A. (2005). Muthi, medicine and witchcraft: Regulating "African Science" in post-Apartheid South Africa? *Social Dynamics, 31*: 211–242.

Azrin, S. T., Goldstein, A. B., & Heinssen, R. K. (2015). Early intervention for psychosis: The recovery after an initial schizophrenia episode project. *Psychiatric Annals, 45*: 548–553.

Baker, R. (1993). The patient's discovery of the psychoanalyst as a new object. *International Journal of Psychoanalysis, 74*: 1223–1233.

Barkan, T., Peled, A., Modai, I., Barak, P., Weizman, A., & Rehavi, M. (2006). Serotonin transporter characteristics in lymphocytes and platelets of male aggressive schizophrenia patients compared to non-aggressive schizophrenia patients. *European Neuropsychopharmacology, 16*: 572–579.

Barrowclough, C., Haddock, G., Lobban, F., Jones, S., Siddle, R., Roberts, C., & Gregg, L. (2006). Group cognitive-behavioural therapy for schizophrenia. *British Journal of Psychiatry, 189*: 527–532.

Baumeister, A. A., & Francis, J. L. (2002). Historical development of the dopamine hypothesis of schizophrenia. *Journal of the History of the Neurosciences, 11*: 265–277.

Bayraktar, G., & Kreutz, M. R. (2018). Neuronal DNA methyltransferases: Epigenetic mediators between synaptic activity and gene expression? *Neuroscientist, 24*: 171–185.

Bell, M., & Bruscato, W. (2002). Object relations deficits in schizophrenia: A cross-cultural comparison between Brazil and the United States. *Journal of Nervous and Mental Disease, 190*: 73–79.

Beraki, S., Aronsson, F., Karlsson, H., Ögren, S. O., & Kristensson, K. (2005). Influenza A virus infection causes alterations in expression of synaptic regulatory genes combined with changes in cognitive and emotional behaviors in mice. *Molecular Psychiatry, 10*: 299–308.

Berson, R. J. (1983). Capgras' syndrome. *American Journal of Psychiatry, 140*: 969–978.

Bhavsar, V., & Bhugra, D. (2008). Religious delusions: Finding meanings in psychosis. *Psychopathology, 41*: 165–172.

Bhugra, D. (2000). Migration and schizophrenia. *Acta Psychiatrica Scandinavica, 102*: 68–73.

Bioque, M., González-Rodríguez, A., Garcia-Rizo, C., Cobo, J., Monreal, J. A., Usall, J., Soria, V., & Labad, J. (2021). Targeting the microbiome-gut-brain axis for improving cognition in schizophrenia and major mood disorders: A narrative review. *Progress in Neuro-Psychopharmacology and Biological Psychiatry, 105*: 110130.

Blokland, G., Grove, J., Chen, C. Y., Cotsapas, C., Tobet, S., Handa, R., Schizophrenia Working Group of the Psychiatric Genomics Consortium, St Clair, D., Lencz, T., Mowry, B. J., Periyasamy, S., Cairns, M. J., Tooney, P. A., Wu, J. Q., Kelly, B., Kirov, G., Sullivan, P. F., Corvin, A., Riley, B. P., Esko, T., [...] Goldstein, J. M. (2021). Sex-dependent shared and nonshared genetic architecture across mood and psychotic disorders. *Biological Psychiatry*, S0006-3223(21)01139-2. Advance online publication.

Bonnigal-Katz, D. (2019). Psychosis therapy project: A psychoanalytic project in the community. *British Journal of Psychotherapy, 35*: 586–589.

Bosnak, R. (1996). *Tracks in the Wilderness of Dreaming*. New York: Delacorte.

Bosnak, R. (2007). *Embodiment: Creative Imagination in Medicine, Art and Travel*. New York: Routledge.

Boydell, J., Van Os, J., Lambri, M., Castle, D., Allardyce, J., McCreadie, R. G., & Murray, R. M. (2003). Incidence of schizophrenia in South-East London between 1965 and 1997. *British Journal of Psychiatry*, *182*: 45–49.

Boyer, L. B. (1961). Provisional evaluation of psycho-analysis with few parameters employed in the treatment of schizophrenia. *International Journal of Psychoanalysis*, *42*: 389–403.

Boyer, L. B. (1971). Psychoanalytic technique in the treatment of certain characterological and schizophrenic disorders. *International Journal of Psychoanalysis*, *52*: 67–85.

Boyer, L. B. (1983). *Regressed Patient*. New York: Jason Aronson.

Brakoulias, V., Starcevic, V., Albert, U., Arumugham, S. S., Bailey, B. E., Belloch, A., & Fineberg, N. A. (2019). Treatments used for obsessive-compulsive disorder—An international perspective. *Human Psychopharmacology*, *34*: e2686.

Brambilla, P., & Tansella, M. (2007). Can neuroimaging studies help us in understanding the biological causes of schizophrenia? *International Review of Psychiatry*, *19*: 313–314.

Braslow, J. T. (1999). History and evidence-based medicine: Lessons from the history of somatic treatments from the 1900s to the 1950s. *Mental Health Services Research*, *1*: 231–240.

Bray, I., Waraich, P., Jones, W., Slater, S., Goldner, E. M., & Somers, J. (2006). Increase in schizophrenia incidence rates: Findings in a Canadian cohort born 1975–1985. *Social Psychiatry and Psychiatric Epidemiology*, *41*: 611–618.

Brazelton, M. T. B., & Greenspan, M. S. I. (2000). *The Irreducible Needs of Children: What Every Child Must Have to Grow, Learn, and Flourish*. Cambridge, MA: Perseus.

Brekke, J. S., & Barrio, C. (1997). Cross-ethnic symptom differences in schizophrenia: The influence of culture and minority status. *Schizophrenia Bulletin*, *23*: 305–316.

Bresnahan, M., Menezes, P., Varma, V., & Susser, E. (2003). Geographical variation in incidence, course and outcome of schizophrenia: A comparison of developing and developed countries. In: R. M. Murray, P. B. Jones, E. Susser, J. van Os, & M. Cannon (Eds.), *The Epidemiology of Schizophrenia* (pp. 18–33). New York: Cambridge University Press.

Brown, A. S., & McGrath, J. J. (2011). The prevention of schizophrenia. *Schizophrenia Bulletin*, *37*: 257–261.

Brown, A. S., & Patterson, P. H. (2011). Maternal infection and schizophrenia: implications for prevention. *Schizophrenia Bulletin*, *37*: 284–290.

Brown, A. S., Schaefer, C. A., Quesenberry, C. P., Shen, L., & Susser, E. S. (2006). No evidence of relation between maternal exposure to herpes simplex virus type 2 and risk of schizophrenia? *American Journal of Psychiatry, 163*: 2178–2180.

Brown, S., Inskip, H., & Barraclough, B. (2000). Causes of the excess mortality of schizophrenia. *British Journal of Psychiatry, 177*: 212–217.

Buckley, L., & Pettit, T. (2007). Supportive therapy for schizophrenia. *Schizophrenia Bulletin, 33*: 859–860.

Buka, S. L., Cannon, T. D., Torrey, E. F., & Yolken, R. H. (2008). Maternal exposure to herpes simplex virus and risk of psychosis among adult offspring. *Biological Psychiatry, 63*: 809–815.

Burnham, D. L., Gibson, R. W., & Gladstone, A. I. (1969). *Schizophrenia and the Need-fear Dilemma*. New York: International Universities Press.

Burns, J. (2007). *The Descent of Madness: Evolutionary Origins of Psychosis and the Social Brain*. New York: Routledge.

Butler, P. D., Susser, E. S., Brown, A. S., Kaufmann, C. A., & Gorman, J. M. (1994). Prenatal nutritional deprivation as a risk factor in schizophrenia: Preclinical evidence. *Neuropsychopharmacology, 11*: 227–235.

Byrne, M., Agerbo, E., Bennedsen, B., Eaton, W. W., & Mortensen, P. B. (2007). Obstetric conditions and risk of first admission with schizophrenia: A Danish national register based study. *Schizophrenia Research, 97*: 51–59.

Cain, A. C., & Cain, B. S. (1964). On replacing a child. *Journal of the American Academy of Child Psychiatry, 3*: 443–456.

Cameron, N. (1961). Introjection, reprojection, and hallucination in the interaction between schizophrenic patient and therapist. *International Journal of Psychoanalysis, 42*: 86–96.

Cancro, R. (1986). General considerations relating to theory in the schizophrenic disorders. In: D. B. Feinsilver (Ed.), *Towards a Comprehensive Model for Schizophrenic Disorders: Psychoanalytic Essays in Memory of Ping-Nie Pao* (pp. 97–107). Hillsdale, NJ: Analytic Press.

Capasso, R. M., Lineberry, T. W., Bostwick, J. M., Decker, P. A., & St. Sauver, J. (2008). Mortality in schizophrenia and schizoaffective disorder: An Olmsted County, Minnesota cohort: 1950–2005. *Schizophrenia Research, 98*: 287–294.

Carré, J. M., McCormick, C. M., & Hariri, A. R. (2011). The social neuroendocrinology of human aggression. *Psychoneuroendocrinology, 36*: 935–944.

Caruso, J. P., & Sheehan, J. P. (2017). Psychosurgery, ethics, and media: A history of Walter Freeman and the lobotomy. *Neurosurgical Focus, 43*: E6.

Cary, B. (1996). *Tales from Jackpine Bob*. Minneapolis, MN: University of Minnesota Press.

Caseras, X., Kirov, G., Kendall, K. M., Rees, E., Legge, S. E., Bracher-Smith, Escott-Price, V., & Murphy, K. (2021). Effects of genomic copy number variants penetrant for schizophrenia on cortical thickness and surface area in healthy individuals: Analysis of the UK Biobank. *British Journal of Psychiatry*, *218*: 104–111.

Casey, D. E., Haupt, D. W., Newcomer, J. W., Henderson, D. C., Sernyak, M. J., Davidson, M., Lindenmayer, J.-P., Manoukian, S. V., Banerji, M. A., Lebovitz, H. E., & Hennekens, C. H. (2004). Antipsychotic-induced weight gain and metabolic abnormalities: Implications for increased mortality in patients with schizophrenia. *Journal of Clinical Psychiatry*, *65*: 4–18.

Castle, D. J., & Morgan, V. (2008). Epidemiology. In: V. Morgan & K. T. Mueser (Eds.), *Clinical Handbook of Schizophrenia* (pp. 14–24). London: Guilford.

Cattane, N., Richetto, J., & Cattaneo, A. (2020). Prenatal exposure to environmental insults and enhanced risk of developing schizophrenia and autism spectrum disorder: Focus on biological pathways and epigenetic mechanisms. *Neuroscience & Biobehavioral Reviews*, *117*: 253–278.

Çetingök, M., Chu, C., & Park, D. (1990). The effect of culture on the sex differences in schizophrenia. *International Journal of Social Psychiatry*, *36*: 272–279.

Chan, S. K. W., Hui, C. L. M., Chang, W. C., Lee, E. H. M., & Chen, E. Y. H. (2019). Ten-year follow up of patients with first-episode schizophrenia spectrum disorder from an early intervention service: Predictors of clinical remission and functional recovery. *Schizophrenia Research*, *204*: 65–71.

Chaudhry, I. B., Husain, N., ur Rahman, R., Husain, M. O., Hamirani, M. M., Kazmi, A., Baig, S., Haddad, P. M., Buch, M. H., Qureshi, I., Mehmood, N., Kiran, T., Fu, B., Afsar, S., & Deakin, B. (2015). A randomised double-blind placebo-controlled 12- week feasibility trial of methotrexate added to treatment as usual in early schizophrenia: Study protocol for a randomised controlled trial. *Trials*, *16*: 9.

Cheng, Y., Chen, C., Lin, C.-P., Chou, K.-H., & Decety, J. (2010). Love hurts: An fMRI study. *NeuroImage*, *51*: 923–929.

Cheniaux, E., Landeira-Fernandez, J., Telles, L. L., Lessa, J. L. M., Dias, A., Duncan, T., & Versiani, M. (2008). Does schizoaffective disorder really exist? A systematic review of the studies that compared schizoaffective disorder with schizophrenia or mood. *Journal of Affective Disorders*, *106*: 209–217.

Chiu, V. W., Ree, M., Janca, A., Iyyalol, R., Dragovic, M., & Waters, F. (2018). Sleep profiles and CBT-I response in schizophrenia and related psychoses. *Psychiatry Research*, *268*: 279–287.

Chused, J. F. (1982). The role of analytic neutrality in the use of the child analyst as a new object. *Journal of the American Psychoanalytic Association, 30*: 3–28.

Chwastiak, L. A., & Tek, C. (2009). The unchanging mortality gap for people with schizophrenia. *Lancet, 374*: 590–592.

Clair, D. S. (2013). Structural and copy number variants in the human genome: Implications for psychiatry. *British Journal of Psychiatry, 202*: 5–6.

Colangeli, R. (2020). Bound together: How psychoanalysis diminishes inter-generational DNA trauma. *American Journal of Psychoanalysis, 80*: 196–218.

Colonna, A. B., & Newman, L. M. (1983). The psychoanalytic literature on siblings. *Psychoanalytic Study of the Child, 38*: 285–309.

Consoli, A. J., Tzaquitzal, M. de los Á. H., & González, A. (2013). Mayan cosmovision and integrative counseling: A case study from Guatemala. In: S. Poyrazli & C. E. Thompson (Eds.), *International Case Studies in Mental Health* (pp. 141–153). Thousand Oaks, CA: Sage.

Conus, P., Cotton, S. M., Francey, S. M., O'Donoghue, B., Schimmelmann, B. G., McGorry, P. D., & Lambert, M. (2017). Predictors of favourable outcome in young people with a first episode psychosis without antipsychotic medication. *Schizophrenia Research, 185*: 130–136.

Cowan, H. R. (2020). Is schizophrenia research relevant during the COVID-19 pandemic? *Schizophrenia Research, 220*: 271–272.

Cullen, A. E., Holmes, S., Pollak, T. A., Blackman, G., Joyce, D. W., Kempton, M. J., Murray, R. M., McGuire, P., & Mondelli, V. (2019). Associations between non-neurological autoimmune disorders and psychosis: A meta-analysis. *Biological Psychiatry, 85*: 35–48.

Dalman, C., Allebeck, P., Gunnell, D., Harrison, G., Kristensson, K., Lewis, G., Lofving, S., Rasmussen, F., Wicks, S., & Karlsson, H. (2008). Infections in the CNS during childhood and the risk of subsequent psychotic illness: A cohort study of more than one million Swedish subjects. *American Journal of Psychiatry, 165*: 59–65.

D'Astous, M., Cottin, S., Roy, M., Picard, C., & Cantin, L. (2013). Bilateral stereotactic anterior capsulotomy for obsessive-compulsive disorder: Long-term follow-up. *Journal of Neurology, Neurosurgery, and Psychiatry, 84*: 1208–1213.

Davenport, S., Hobson, R., & Margison, F. (2000). Treatment development in psychodynamic-interpersonal psychotherapy (Hobson's "Conversational Model") for chronic treatment resistant schizophrenia: Two single case studies. *British Journal of Psychotherapy, 16*: 287–302.

Davis, J. M., & Leucht, S. (2008). Has research informed us on the practical drug treatment of schizophrenia? *Schizophrenia Bulletin, 34*: 403–405.

De Luca, V., Zai, G., Tharmalingam, S., de Bartolomeis, A., Wong, G., & Kennedy, J. L. (2006). Association study between the novel functional polymorphism of the serotonin transporter gene and suicidal behaviour in schizophrenia. *European Neuropsychopharmacology, 16*: 268–271.

De Masi, F. (2020). Psychosis and analytic therapy: A complex relationship. *International Journal of Psychoanalysis, 101*: 152–168.

Dean, B., Hussain, T., Scarr, E., Pavey, G., & Copolov, D. L. (2001). Extended treatment with typical and atypical antipsychotic drugs: Differential effects on the densities of dopamine D-sub-2-like and GABA-sub(A) receptors in rat striatum. *Life Sciences, 69*: 1257–1268.

Dean, B., Pavey, G., Thomas, D., & Scarr, E. (2006). Cortical serotonin-sub (7, 1D) and -sub(1F) receptors: Effects of schizophrenia, suicide and antipsychotic drug treatment. *Schizophrenia Research, 88*: 265–274.

Dean, K., Bramon, E., & Murray, R. M. (2003). The causes of schizophrenia: Neurodevelopment and other risk factors. *Journal of Psychiatric Practice, 9*: 442–454.

Devinsky, O., & Lai, G. (2008). Spirituality and religion in epilepsy. *Epilepsy & Behavior, 12*: 636–643.

Dickerson, F., Boronow, J., Stallings, C., Origoni, A., & Yolken, R. (2007). Toxoplasma gondii in individuals with schizophrenia: Association with clinical and demographic factors and with mortality. *Schizophrenia Bulletin, 33*: 737–740.

Dickerson, F., Kirkpatrick, B., Boronow, J., Stallings, C., Origoni, A., & Yolken, R. (2006). Deficit schizophrenia: Association with serum antibodies to cytomegalovirus. *Schizophrenia Bulletin, 32*: 396–400.

Dickerson, F., Severance, E., & Yolken, R. (2017). The microbiome, immunity, and schizophrenia and bipolar disorder. *Brain, Behavior, and Immunity, 62*: 46–52.

Dickson, H., Hedges, E. P., Ma, S. Y., Cullen, A. E., MacCabe, J. H., Kempton, M. J., Downs, J., & Laurens, K. R. (2020). Academic achievement and schizophrenia: A systematic meta-analysis. *Psychological Medicine, 50*: 1949–1965.

Dion, G. L., & Dellario, D. (1988). Symptom subtypes in persons institution-alized with schizophrenia: Comparison of demographics, outcome and functional skills. *Rehabilitation Psychology, 33*: 95–104.

Divac, N., Prostran, M., Jakovcevski, I., & Cerovac, N. (2014). Second-generation antipsychotics and extrapyramidal adverse effects. *BioMed Research International*: 656370.

Dorpat, T. L. (1976). Structural conflict and object relations conflict. *Journal of the American Psychoanalytic Association, 24*: 855–874.

dosReis, S., Johnson, E., Steinwachs, D., Rohde, C., Skinner, E. A., Fahey, M., & Lehman, A. F. (2008). Antipsychotic treatment patterns and hospitalizations among adults with schizophrenia. *Schizophrenia Research, 101*: 304–311.

Downing, D. L., & Mills, J. (2018). *Outpatient Treatment of Psychosis: Psychodynamic Approaches to Evidence-Based Practice*. New York: Routledge.

Duggal, H. S., Jagadheesan, K., & Nizamie, S. H. (2002). Acute onset of schizophrenia following autocastration. *Canadian Journal of Psychiatry. Revue Canadienne De Psychiatrie, 47*: 283–284.

Dully, H., & Fleming, C. (2007). *My Lobotomy*. New York: Crown.

Dykxhoorn, J., Hollander, A.-C., Lewis, G., Magnusson, C., Dalman, C., & Kirkbride, J. B. (2019). Risk of schizophrenia, schizoaffective, and bipolar disorders by migrant status, region of origin, and age-at-migration: A national cohort study of 18 million people. *Psychological Medicine, 49*: 2354–2363.

Edwards, F. S. (1984). Amafufunyana spirit possession: A report on some recent developments. *Religion in Southern Africa, 5*: 3–16.

Eecke, W. V. (2019). How does psychoanalysis work with persons afflicted by schizophrenia? *Journal of Psychology & Psychotherapy, 9*: 1–5.

Ekstein, R. (1966). *Children of Time and Space, of Action and Impulse: Clinical Studies on the Psychoanalytic Treatment of Severely Disturbed Children*. New York: Appleton-Century-Crofts.

Ellenbroek, B., & Youn, J. (2016). The genetic basis of behavior. In: B. Ellenbroek & J. Youn (Eds.), *Gene-Environment Interactions in Psychiatry* (pp. 19–46). San Diego, CA: Academic Press.

Elwin, V. (1955). *The Religion of an Indian Tribe*. Oxford: Oxford University Press.

Emde, R. N. (1981). Changing models of infancy and the nature of early development: Remodeling the foundation. *Journal of the American Psychoanalytic Association, 29*: 179–218.

Emde, R. N. (1988a). Development terminable and interminable: I. Innate and motivational factors from infancy. *International Journal of Psychoanalysis, 69*: 23–42.

Emde, R. N. (1988b). Development terminable and interminable: II. Recent psychoanalytic theory and therapeutic considerations. *International Journal of Psychoanalysis, 69*: 283–296.

Enger, C., Weatherby, L., Reynolds, R. F., Glasser, D. B., & Walker, A. M. (2004). Serious cardiovascular events and mortality among patients with schizophrenia. *Journal of Nervous and Mental Disease, 192*: 19–27.

Ensink, K., & Robertson, B. (1996). Indigenous categories of distress and dysfunction in South African Xhosa children and adolescents as described by indigenous healers. *Transcultural Psychiatric Research Review, 33*: 137–172.

Erikson, E. H. (1950). *Identity and the Life Cycle*. New York: W. W. Norton.

Eyles, D. W. (2021). How do established developmental risk-factors for schizophrenia change the way the brain develops? *Translational Psychiatry, 11*: 1–15.

Fairbairn, W. R. D. (1952). *Psychoanalytic Studies of the Personality*. London: Routledge & Kegan Paul.

Fakra, E., Salgado-Pineda, P., Delaveau, P., Hariri, A. R., & Blin, O. (2008). Neural bases of different cognitive strategies for facial affect processing in schizophrenia. *Schizophrenia Research, 100*: 191–205.

Fan, J. B., & Sklar, P. (2005). Meta-analysis reveals association between serotonin transporter gene STin2 VNTR polymorphism and schizophrenia. *Molecular Psychiatry, 10*: 928–938.

Fatemi, S. H., Reutiman, T. J., Folsom, T. D., Huang, H., Oishi, K., Mori, S., Smee, D. F., Pearce, D. A., Winter, C., Sohr, R., & Juckel, G. (2008). Maternal infection leads to abnormal gene regulation and brain atrophy in mouse offspring: implications for genesis of neurodevelopmental disorders. *Schizophrenia Research, 99*: 56–70.

Fearon, P., Kirkbride, J. B., Morgan, C., Dazzan, P., Morgan, K., Lloyd, T., Hutchinson, G., Tarrant, J., Fung, W. L. A., Holloway, J., Mallett, R., Harrison, G., Leff, J., Jones, P. B., & Murray, R. M. (2006). Incidence of schizophrenia and other psychoses in ethnic minority groups: Results from the MRC AESOP Study. *Psychological Medicine, 36*: 1541–1550.

Fenichel, O. (1945). *The Psychoanalytic Theory of Neurosis*. New York: W. W. Norton.

Ferenczi, S., & Jones, E. (1916). *Contributions to Psycho-analysis*. Boston, MA: Richard G. Badger.

Fierini, F., Moretti, D., & Ballerini, A. (2020). Psychosis spectrum disorders during and after the COVID-19 pandemic: Warning signs of "stress incubation." *Psychiatry Research, 291*: 113291.

Findlay, L. J. (2012). *Decision-Making Processes and Health Behaviors among Adults Diagnosed with Schizophrenia*. Ann Arbor, MI: ProQuest Information & Learning.

Fisch, R. Z. (1992). Psychosis precipitated by marriage: A culture-bound syndrome? *British Journal of Medical Psychology, 65*: 385–391.

Fischmann, T. (2016). Dreams, unconscious fantasies and epigenetics. In: S. Weigel & G. Scharbert (Eds.), *A Neuro-psychoanalytical Dialogue for*

Bridging Freud and the Neurosciences (pp. 91–105). Cham, Switzerland: Springer International.

Flegr, J., & Kuba, R. (2016). The relation of toxoplasma infection and sexual attraction to fear, danger, pain, and submissiveness. *Evolutionary Psychology*, *14*: 1–10.

Fonseca, L., Diniz, E., Mendonça, G., Malinowski, F., Mari, J., & Gadelha, A. (2020). Schizophrenia and COVID-19: Risks and recommendations. *Brazilian Journal of Psychiatry*, *42*: 236–238.

Forman, M. (1975). *One Flew Over the Cuckoo's Nest*. Warner Studios.

Fornito, A., Yücel, M., Wood, S. J., Adamson, C., Velakoulis, D., Saling, M. M., McGory, P. D., & Pantelis, C. (2008). Surface-based morphometry of the anterior cingulate cortex in first episode schizophrenia. *Human Brain Mapping*, *29*: 478–489.

Fors, B. M., Isacson, D., Bingefors, K., & Widerlöv, B. (2007). Mortality among persons with schizophrenia in Sweden: An epidemiological study. *Nordic Journal of Psychiatry*, *61*: 252–259.

Foussias, G., & Remington, G. (2010). Antipsychotics and schizophrenia: From efficacy and effectiveness to clinical decision-making. *Canadian Journal of Psychiatry. Revue Canadienne De Psychiatrie*, *55*: 117–125.

Frankle, W. G., Lombardo, I., Kegeles, L. S., Slifstein, M., Martin, J. H., Huang, Y., Hwang, D.-R., Reich, E., Cangiano, C., Gil, R., Laruelle, M., & Abi-Dargham, A. (2006). Serotonin 1A receptor availability in patients with schizophrenia and schizo-affective disorder: A positron emission tomography imaging study with [^{11}C] WAY 100635. *Psychopharmacology*, *189*: 155–164.

Frantzis, B. K. (1993). *Opening the Energy Gates of Your Body*. Berkeley, CA: North Atlantic.

Freud, A. (1954). *The Writings of Anna Freud, Vol. 4*. New York: International Universities Press.

Freud, S. (1911c). Psycho-analytic notes on an autobiographical account of a case of paranoia (Dementia Paranoides). *S. E.*, *12*: 1–82. London: Hogarth.

Freud, S. (1914d). On the history of the psycho-analytic movement. *S. E.*, *14*: 1–66. London: Hogarth.

Freud, S. (1915e). The unconscious. *S. E.* , *14*: 159–215. London: Hogarth.

Freud, S. (1923b). *The Ego and the Id*. *S. E.*, *19*: 1–66. London: Hogarth.

Freud, S. (1924b). Neurosis and psychosis. *S. E.*, *19*: 147–154. London: Hogarth.

Freud, S. (1924e). The loss of reality in neurosis and psychosis. *S. E.*, *19*: 181–188. London: Hogarth.

Freud, S. (1950a). A project for a scientific psychology. *S. E.*, *1*: 283–397. London: Hogarth.

Fröhlich, F., & Lustenberger, C. (2020). Neuromodulation of sleep rhythms in schizophrenia: Towards the rational design of non-invasive brain stimulation. *Schizophrenia Research, 221*: 71–80.

Fromm-Reichmann, F. (1939). Transference problems in schizophrenics. *Psychoanalytic Quarterly, 8*: 412–426.

Fromm-Reichmann, F. (1959). *Psychoanalysis and Psychotherapy: Selected Papers of Frieda Fromm-Reichmann.* Chicago, IL: University of Chicago Press.

Fu, S., Czajkowski, N., & Torgalsbøen, A. K. (2019). Cognitive, work, and social outcomes in fully recovered first-episode schizophrenia: On and off antipsychotic medication. *Psychiatry, 82*: 42–56.

Fuchs, S. H. (1937). On introjection. *International Journal of Psychoanalysis, 18*: 269–293.

Furnham, A., & Wong, L. (2007). A cross-cultural comparison of British and Chinese beliefs about the causes, behaviour manifestations and treatment of schizophrenia. *Psychiatry Research, 151*: 123–138.

Garfield, D., & Mackler, D. (2013). *Beyond Medication: Therapeutic Engagement and the Recovery from Psychosis.* New York: Routledge.

Garver, D. L., Holcomb, J. A., & Christensen, J. D. (2000). Heterogeneity of response to antipsychotics from multiple disorders in the schizophrenia spectrum. *Journal of Clinical Psychiatry, 61*: 964–974.

Gault, J. M., Davis, R., Cascella, N. G, Saks, E. R., & Corripio-Collado, I. (2018). Approaches to neuromodulation for schizophrenia. *Journal of Neurology, Neurosurgery & Psychiatry, 89*: 777–787.

Gazdag, G., & Ungvari, G. S. (2019). Electroconvulsive therapy: 80 years old and still going strong. *World Journal of Psychiatry, 9*: 1–6.

Gearon, J. S., Bellack, A. S., Rachbeisel, J., & Dixon, L. (2001). Drug-use behavior and correlates in people with schizophrenia. *Addictive Behaviors, 26*: 51–61.

Gibbs, P. L. (2007). The primacy of psychoanalytic intervention in recovery from the psychoses and schizophrenias. *Journal of the American Academy of Psychoanalysis and Dynamic Psychiatry, 35*: 287–312.

Gibson, E. L., Barr, S., & Jeanes, Y. M. (2013). Habitual fat intake predicts memory function in younger women. *Frontiers in Human Neuroscience, 7*: 838.

Gil, A., Gama, C. S., de Jesus, D. R., Lobato, M. I., Zimmer, M., & Belmonte-de-Abreu, P. (2009). The association of child abuse and neglect with adult disability in schizophrenia and the prominent role of physical neglect. *Child Abuse & Neglect, 33*: 618–624.

Gilmore, J. H. (2010). Understanding what causes schizophrenia: A developmental perspective. *American Journal of Psychiatry, 167*: 8–10.

Gilmour, G., Dix, S., Fellini, L., Gastambide, F., Plath, N., Steckler, T., Talpos, J., & Tricklebank, M. (2012). NMDA receptors, cognition and schizophrenia—testing the validity of the NMDA receptor hypofunction hypothesis. *Neuropharmacology, 62*: 1401–1412.

Giovacchini, P. L. (1969). The influence of interpretation upon schizophrenic patients. *International Journal of Psychoanalysis, 50*: 179–186.

Giovacchini, P. L. (1972). Interpretation and definition of the analytic setting. In P. Giovacchini (Ed.), *Tactics and Techniques in Psychoanalytic Therapy.* (pp. 65–70). Northvale, NJ: Jason Aronson

Giovacchini, P. L., & Boyer, B. L. (1980). *Psychoanalytic Treatment of Schizophrenic Borderline and Characterological Disorders.* New York: Jason Aronson.

Girdler, S. J., Confino, J. E., & Woesner, M. E. (2019). Exercise as a treatment for schizophrenia: A review. *Psychopharmacology Bulletin, 49*: 56–69.

Glass, J. (1985). *Delusion: Internal Dimensions of Political Life.* Chicago, IL: University of Chicago Press.

Gold, C. (2015). Dose and effect in CBT for schizophrenia. *British Journal of Psychiatry, 207*: 269–273.

Gomes, F. V., & Grace, A. A. (2018). Cortical dopamine dysregulation in schizophrenia and its link to stress. *Brain: A Journal of Neurology, 141*: 1897–1899.

Gong, H., & Xu, X. (2017). The epigenetics of brain aging and psychiatric disorders. In: D. H. Yasui, J. Peedicayil, & D. R. Grayson (Eds.), *Neuropsychiatric Disorders and Epigenetics* (pp. 141–162). San Diego, CA: Academic Press.

González de Chávez, M. (2009). Treatment of psychoses before the twentieth century. In: Y. O. Alanen, M. González de Chávez, A.-L. S. Silver, & B. Martindale (Eds.), *Psychotherapeutic Approaches to Schizophrenic Psychoses: Past, Present and Future* (pp. 10–22). New York: Routledge.

Gonzalez-Flores, B. L. (2020). *Impact of Independent Exercise on Recovery, Well-being, and Motivation among Individuals with Schizophrenia.* Ann Arbor, MI: ProQuest Information & Learning.

Gorman, J. M. (2016). Combining psychodynamic psychotherapy and pharmacotherapy. *Psychodynamic Psychiatry, 44*: 183–209.

Gössler, R., Vesely, C., & Friedrich, M. H. (2002). Autocastration of a young schizophrenic man. *Psychiatrische Praxis, 29*: 214–217.

Gottdiener, W. H. (2006). Individual psychodynamic psychotherapy of schizophrenia: Empirical evidence for the practicing clinician. *Psychoanalytic Psychology, 23*: 583–589.

Gray, L., Scarr, E., & Dean, B. (2006). Serotonin 1a receptor and associated G-protein activation schizophrenia and bipolar disorder. *Psychiatry Research, 143*: 111–120.

Green, M., & Solnit, A. J. (1964). Reactions to a threatened loss of a child: A vulnerable child syndrome. *Pediatrics, 34*: 58–66.

Green, M. F., Horan, W. P., & Lee, J. (2019). Nonsocial and social cognition in schizophrenia: Current evidence and future directions. *World Psychiatry, 18*: 146–161.

Greenacre, P. (1970). The transitional object and the fetish with special reference to the role of illusion. *International Journal of Psychoanalysis, 51*: 447–456.

Greenspan, S. I. (1990). *The Development of the Ego: Implications for Personality Theory, Psychopathology, and the Psychotherapeutic Process.* Madison, CT: International Universities Press.

Greenspan, S. I., & Benderly, B. L. (1997). *The Growth of the Mind and the Endangered Origins of Intelligence.* Cambridge, MA: Perseus.

Grignon, S., & Trottier, M. (2005). Capgras syndrome in the modern era: Self misidentification on an ID Picture. *Canadian Journal of Psychiatry, 50*: 74–75.

Grotstein, J. S. (1986). Schizophrenic personality disorder: "… and if I should die before I wake." In: D. Feinsilver (Ed.), *Towards a Comprehensive Model for Schizophrenic Disorders.* Hillsdale, NJ: Routledge.

Grotstein, J. S. (1990a). Nothingness, meaninglessness, chaos, and the "black hole": II The black hole. *Contemporary Psychoanalysis, 26*: 377–407.

Grotstein, J. S. (1990b). The "black hole" as the basic psychotic experience: Some newer psychoanalytic and neuroscience perspectives on psychosis. *Journal of the American Academy of Psychoanalysis, 18*: 29–46.

Grotstein, J. S. (1991). Nothingness, meaninglessness, chaos, and the "black hole": III Self- and interactional regulation and the background presence of primary identification. *Contemporary Psychoanalysis, 27*: 1–33.

Grotstein, J. S. (2001). A rationale for the psychoanalytically informed psychotherapy of schizophrenia and other psychoses: Towards the concept of "rehabilitative psychoanalysis." In: P. Williams (Ed.), *A Language for Psychosis: Psychoanalysis of Psychotic States* (pp. 9–26). Hoboken, NJ: John Wiley & Sons.

Grotstein, J. S. (2003). Towards the concept of "rehabilitative psychoanalytic psychotherapy" in the treatment of schizophrenia. In: A. Grispini (Ed.), *Preventive Strategies for Schizophrenic Disorders: Basic Principles, Opportunities and Limits* (pp. 350–365). Rome: Giovanni Fioriti Editore.

Gründer, G., & Cumming, P. (2016). The dopamine hypothesis of schizophrenia: Current status. In: T. Abel & T. Nickl-Jockschat (Eds.), *The Neurobiology of Schizophrenia* (pp. 109–124). San Diego, CA: Elsevier Academic Press.

Guadalupe, L. A. O., Miranda, R. T., Soto Prada, K.-J., Borrero, T. C., Cortes Peña, O. F., Scarpati, M. P., & Ucrós Campo, M. M. (2017). Incidencia de mindfulness y Qi Gong sobre el estado de salud, bienestar psicológico, satisfacción vital y estrés laboral. *Revista Colombiana de Psicología, 26*: 99–113.

Gulsuner, S., & McClellan, J. M. (2015). Copy number variation in schizophrenia. *Neuropsychopharmacology, 40*: 252–254.

Gur, R. E., Loughead, J., Kohler, C. G., Elliott, M. A., Lesko, K., Ruparel, K., Wolf, D. H., Bilker, W. B., & Gur, R. C. (2007). Limbic activation associated with misidentification of fearful faces and flat affect in schizophrenia. *Archives of General Psychiatry, 64*: 1356–1366.

Gürel, Ç., Kuşçu, G. C., Yavaşoğlu, A., & Biray Avcı, Ç. (2020). The clues in solving the mystery of major psychosis: The epigenetic basis of schizophrenia and bipolar disorder. *Neuroscience & Biobehavioral Reviews, 113*: 51–61.

Gyuris, J. (2011). Psychiatric aspects of autocastration. *Psychiatria Hungarica: A Magyar Pszichiatriai Tarsasag Tudomanyos Folyoirata, 26*: 128–131.

Hadar, R., Bikovski, L., Soto-Montenegro, M. L., Schimke, J., Maier, P., Ewing, S., & Winter, C. (2018). Early neuromodulation prevents the development of brain and behavioral abnormalities in a rodent model of schizophrenia. *Molecular Psychiatry, 23*: 943–951.

Hagen, C. A., & Schokking, I. D. (1990). Hysteria and conversion in the Ojibway patient: Cross-cultural psychiatry for the family physician. *Canadian Family Physician, 36*: 275–279.

Hagiwara, H., Fujita, Y., Ishima, T., Kunitachi, S., Shirayama, Y., Iyo, M., & Hashimoto, K. (2008). Phencyclidine-induced cognitive deficits in mice are improved by subsequent subchronic administration of the antipsychotic drug perospirone: Role of serotonin 5-HT-sub(1A) receptors. *European Neuropsychopharmacology, 18*: 448–454.

Hallowell, A. I. (1936). Psychic stresses and culture patterns. *American Journal of Psychiatry, 92*: 1291–1310.

Hartmann, H. (1939). Ich-psychologie und anpassungsproblem. *Internationale Zeitschrift Für Psychoanalyse und Imago, 24*: 62–135.

Hartmann, H. (1954). Contribution to the metapsychology of schizophrenia. *Psychoanalytic Study of the Child, 8*: 177–198.

Hashimoto, T., Bazmi, H. H., Mirnics, K., Wu, Q., Sampson, A. R., & Lewis, D. A. (2008). Conserved regional patterns of GABA-related transcript expression in the neocortex of subjects with schizophrenia. *American Journal of Psychiatry*, *165*: 479–489.

Healy, D. (2006). Neuroleptics and mortality: A 50-year cycle: Invited commentary on schizophrenia, neuroleptic medication and mortality. *British Journal of Psychiatry*, *188*: 128.

Heckel, T., Singh, A., Gschwind, A., Reymond, A., & Certa, U. (2015). Genetic variations in the macaca fascicularis genome related to biomedical research. In: J. Bluemel, S. Korte, E. Schenck, & G. F. Weinbauer (Eds.), *The Nonhuman Primate in Nonclinical Drug Development and Safety Assessment* (pp. 53–64). San Diego, CA: Academic Press.

Hendrick, I. (1928). Encephalitis lethargica and the interpretation of mental disease. *American Journal of Psychiatry*, *7*: 989–1014.

Heng, H. H. (2017). The genomic landscape of cancers. In: B. Ujvari, B. Roche, & F. Thomas (Eds.), *Ecology and Evolution of Cancer* (pp. 69–86). San Diego, CA: Academic Press.

Henssler, J., Brandt, L., Müller, M., Liu, S., Montag, C., Sterzer, P., & Heinz, A. (2020). Migration and schizophrenia: Meta-analysis and explanatory framework. *European Archives of Psychiatry and Clinical Neuroscience*, *270*: 325–335.

Hilker, R., Helenius, D., Fagerlund, B., Skytthe, A., Christensen, K., Werge, T. M., Nordentoft, M., & Glenthøj, B. (2018). Heritability of schizophrenia and schizophrenia spectrum based on the nationwide Danish twin register. *Biological Psychiatry*, *83*: 492–498.

Hiraoka, A., Kobayashi, H., Shimono, F., & Ohsuga, M. (1997). Effects of Kai-Gou (air-ball handling): A Qi-Gong strategy, on the biofeedback training for enhancement of the electroencephalographic α-activity. *Japanese Journal of Biofeedback Research*, *24*: 74–78.

Hodge, J. M., Coghill, A. E., Kim, Y., Bender, N., Smith-Warner, S. A., Gapstur, S., & Egan, K. M. (2021). Toxoplasma gondii infection and the risk of adult glioma in two prospective studies. *International Journal of Cancer*, *148*: 2449–2456.

Hoeffding, L. K., Rosengren, A., Thygesen, J. H., Schmock, H., Werge, T., & Hansen, T. (2017). Evaluation of shared genetic susceptibility loci between autoimmune diseases and schizophrenia based on genome-wide association studies. *Nordic Journal of Psychiatry*, *71*: 20–25.

Hong, J., & Bang, M. (2020). Anti-inflammatory strategies for schizophrenia: A review of evidence for therapeutic applications and drug repurposing. *Clinical Psychopharmacology and Neuroscience*, *18*: 10–24.

Høyersten, J. G. (1996). Possessed! Some historical, psychiatric and current moments of demonic possession. *Tidsskrift for Den Norske Laegeforening: Tidsskrift for Praktisk Medicin, Ny Raekke, 116*: 3602–3606.

Hua, M., Peng, Y., Zhou, Y., Qin, W., Yu, C., & Liang, M. (2020). Disrupted pathways from limbic areas to thalamus in schizophrenia highlighted by whole-brain resting-state effective connectivity analysis. *Progress in Neuro-Psychopharmacology and Biological Psychiatry, 99*: 109837.

Huang, T. (2019). Copy number variations in tumors. In: P. Boffetta & P. Hainaut (Eds.), *Encyclopedia of Cancer* (pp. 444–451). San Diego, CA: Academic Press.

Hutchinson, G., Bhugra, D., Mallett, R., Burnett, R., Corridan, B., & Leff, J. (1999). Fertility and marital rates in first-onset schizophrenia. *Social Psychiatry and Psychiatric Epidemiology, 34*: 617–621.

Hwang, J.-Y., Aromolaran, K. A., & Zukin, R. S. (2017). The emerging field of epigenetics in neurodegeneration and neuroprotection. *Nature Reviews Neuroscience, 18*: 347–361.

Hwang, W.-C. (2007). Qi-gong psychotic reaction in a Chinese American woman. *Culture, Medicine and Psychiatry, 31*: 547–560.

Iannitelli, A., Parnanzone, S., Pizziconi, G., Riccobono, G., & Pacitti, F. (2019). Psychodynamically oriented psychopharmacotherapy: Towards a necessary synthesis. *Frontiers in Human Neuroscience, 13*: 15.

İpçi, K., Yıldız, M., İncedere, A., Kiras, F., Esen, D., & Gürcan, M. B. (2020). Subjective recovery in patients with schizophrenia and related factors. *Community Mental Health Journal, 56*: 1180–1187.

Jacobson, E. (1964). *The Self and the Object World*. Oxford: International Universities Press.

Janssen, I., Krabbendam, L., Bak, M., Hanssen, M., Vollebergh, W., de Graaf, R., & van Os, J. (2004). Childhood abuse as a risk factor for psychotic experiences. *Acta Psychiatrica Scandinavica, 109*: 38–45.

Jauhur, S., McKenna, P. J., Radua, J., Fung, E., Salvador, R., & Laws, K. R. (2014). Cognitive-behavioural therapy for the symptoms of schizophrenia: Systematic review and meta-analysis with examination of potential bias. *British Journal of Psychiatry, 204*: 20–29.

Jentsch, J. D., & Roth, R. H. (1999). The neuropsychopharmacology of phency-clidine: From NMDA receptor hypofunction to the dopamine hypothesis of schizophrenia. *Neuropsychopharmacology, 20*: 201–225.

Jia, J., Shen, J., Liu, F.-H., Wong, H. K., Yang, X.-J., Wu, Q.-J., Zhang, H., Wang, H.-N., Tan, Q.-R., & Zhang, Z.-J. (2019). Effectiveness of electroacupuncture and electroconvulsive therapy as additional treatment in hospitalized patients with schizophrenia: A retrospective controlled study. *Frontiers in Psychology, 10*: 1–9.

Jobe, E. M., & Zhao, X. (2017). DNA methylation and adult neurogenesis. *Brain Plasticity, 3*: 5–26.

Johnson, B., & Flores Mosri, D. (2016). The neuropsychoanalytic approach: Using neuroscience as the basic science of psychoanalysis. *Frontiers in Psychology, 7*: 1459.

Joukamaa, M., Heliövaara, M., Knekt, P., Aromaa, A., Raitasalo, R., & Lehtinen, V. (2006). Schizophrenia, neuroleptic medication and mortality. *British Journal of Psychiatry, 188*: 122–127.

Joyal, C. C., Hallé, P., Lapierre, D., & Hodgins, S. (2003). Drug abuse and/or dependence and better neuropsychological performance in patients with schizophrenia. *Schizophrenia Research, 63*: 297–299.

Juckel, G., & Hoffmann, K. (2018). The Indian Ayurveda medicine—a meaningful supplement to psychiatric treatment? *Der Nervenarzt, 89*: 999–1008.

Jung, C. G. (1925). The content of the psychoses. In: J. S. Van Teslaar (Ed.), *An Outline of Psychoanalysis* (pp. 255–271). New York: Modern Library.

Kane, J. M., & Leucht, S. (2008). Unanswered questions in schizophrenia clinical trials. *Schizophrenia Bulletin, 34*: 302–309.

Kapelski, P., Hauser, J., Dmitrzak-Weglarz, M., Skibinska, M., Slopien, A., Kaczmarkiewicz-Fass, M., Rajewska, A., Gattner, K., & Czerski, P. M. (2006). Brak asocjacji pomiedzy polimorfizmem insercyjno-delecyjnym promoto-rowego odcinka genu transportera serotoniny a schizofrenia. *Psychiatria Polska, 40*: 925–935.

Kapsambelis, V. (2019). Psychoanalytic approaches to psychotic disorders in a public mental health system. *British Journal of Psychotherapy, 35*: 577–585.

Kastrup, M. C., Báez-Ramos, A., Moodley, R., Lubin, D. B., Akram, S., & Justin, M. (2008). Case incident 10: Counseling for transition trauma and health concerns. In: N. Arthur & P. Pedersen (Eds.), *Case Incidents in Counseling for International Transitions* (pp. 151–167). Alexandria, VA: American Counseling Association.

Kee, K. S., Horan, W. P., Wynn, J. K., Mintz, J., & Green, M. F. (2006). An analysis of categorical perception of facial emotion in schizophrenia. *Schizophrenia Research, 87*: 228–237.

Kelly, D. L., Rowland, L. M., Patchan, K. M., Sullivan, K., Earl, A., Raley, H., Lui, F., Feldman, S., & McMahon, R. P. (2016). Schizophrenia clinical symptom differences in women vs men with and without a history of childhood physical abuse. *Child and Adolescent Psychiatry and Mental Health, 10*: 5.

Kernberg, O. F. (1966). Structural derivatives of object relationships. *International Journal of Psychoanalysis, 47*: 236–253.

Kernberg, O. F. (1970). A psychoanalytic classification of character pathology. *Journal of the American Psychoanalytic Association, 18*: 800–822.

Kernberg, O. F. (1975). *Borderline Conditions and Pathological Narcissism.* New York: Jason Aronson.

Kernberg, O. F. (1976). *Object Relations Theory and Clinical Psychoanalysis.* New York: Jason Aronson.

Kernberg, O. F. (1984). *Severe Personality Disorders: Psychotherapeutic Strategies.* New Haven, CT: Yale University Press.

Kesey, K. (1962). *One Flew Over the Cuckoo's Nest.* New York: Viking.

Keshavan, M., Lizano, P., & Prasad, K. (2020). The synaptic pruning hypothesis of schizophrenia: Promises and challenges. *World Psychiatry, 19*: 110–111.

Kessler, R. J., & Zellner, M. (2019). Developments in metapsychology: Contributions to neuropsychoanalytic engagement with Freud, and new links to Lacan. *Neuropsychoanalysis, 21*: 1–2.

Khandaker, G. M., Zimbron, J., Dalman, C., Lewis, G., & Jones, P. B. (2012). Childhood infection and adult schizophrenia: A meta-analysis of population-based studies. *Schizophrenia Research, 139*: 161–168.

Kim, H., Kim, D., & Kim, S. H. (2018). Association of types of delusions and hallucinations with childhood abuse and neglect among inpatients with schizophrenia in South Korea: A preliminary study. *Psychosis: Psychological, Social and Integrative Approaches, 10*: 208–212.

Kitcher, P., & Wilkes, K. V. (1988). What is Freud's metapsychology? *Proceedings of the Aristotelian Society, Supplementary Volumes, 62*: 101–137.

Klein, G. (1976). Psychoanalytic theory: an exploration of essentials. New York: International Universities Press.

Klein, M. (1946). Notes on some schizoid mechanisms. *International Journal of Psychoanalysis, 27*: 99–110.

Kline, J., Becker, J., & Giese, C. (1992). Psychodynamic interventions revisited: Options for the treatment of schizophrenia. *Psychotherapy: Theory, Research, Practice, Training, 29*: 366–377.

Knight, J. G. (1982). Dopamine-receptor-stimulating autoantibodies: A possible cause of schizophrenia. *Lancet, 2*: 1073–1076.

Knight, J. G., Menkes, D. B., Highton, J., & Adams, D. D. (2007). Rationale for a trial of immunosuppressive therapy in acute schizophrenia. *Molecular Psychiatry, 12*: 424–431.

Koch, E., Rosenthal, B., Lundquist, A., Chen, C.-H., & Kauppi, K. (2020). Interactome overlap between schizophrenia and cognition. *Schizophrenia Research, 222*: 167–174.

Kohler, C. G., Loughead, J., Ruparel, K., Indersmitten, T., Barrett, F. S., Gur, R. E., & Gur, R. C. (2008). Brain activation during eye gaze discrimination in stable schizophrenia. *Schizophrenia Research, 99*: 286–293.

Kohut, H. (1971). *The Analysis of the Self: A Systematic Approach to the Psychoanalytic Treatment of Narcissistic Personality Disorders*. Chicago, IL: University of Chicago Press.

Kortegaard, H. M. (1993). Music therapy in the psychodynamic treatment of schizophrenia. In: M. H. Heal & T. Wigram (Eds.), *Music Therapy in Health and Education* (pp. 55–65). London: Jessica Kingsley.

Kosugi, D., & Fujita, K. (2001). Infants' recognition of causality: Discrimination between inanimate objects and people. *Psychologia: An International Journal of Psychology in the Orient, 44*: 31–45.

Kozloff, N., Mulsant, B. H., Stergiopoulos, V., & Voineskos, A. N. (2020). The COVID-19 global pandemic: Implications for people with schizophrenia and related disorders. *Schizophrenia Bulletin, 46*: 752–757.

Kraguljac, N. V., Anthony, T., Morgan, C. J., Jindal, R. D., Burger, M. S., & Lahti, A. C. (2020). White matter integrity, duration of untreated psychosis, and antipsychotic treatment response in medication-naïve first-episode psychosis patients. *Molecular Psychiatry* (May 12): 1–10.

Krippner, S. (2019). Shamanism and dreams. In: R. J. Hoss & R. P. Gongloff (Eds.), *Dreams: Understanding Biology, Psychology, and Culture., Vol. 2* (pp. 706–710). Santa Barbara, CA: Greenwood.

Krogmann, A., Peters, L., von Hardenberg, L., Bödeker, K., Nöhles, V. B., & Correll, C. U. (2019). Keeping up with the therapeutic advances in schizophrenia: A review of novel and emerging pharmacological entities. *CNS Spectrums, 24*: 38–69.

Kroll, J. L. (2007). New directions in the conceptualization of psychotic disorders. *Current Opinion in Psychiatry, 20*: 573–577.

Kuijpers, H. J. H., van der Heijden, F. M. M. A., Tuinier, S., & Verhoeven, W. M. A. (2007). Meditation-induced psychosis. *Psychopathology, 40*: 461–464.

Kumar, V., Vajawat, B., & Rao, N. P. (2020). Frontal GABA in schizophrenia: A meta-analysis of 1h-mrs studies. *World Journal of Biological Psychiatry, 22*: 1–13.

Kurihara, T., Kato, M., Reverger, R., & Tirta, I. G. R. (2006). Beliefs about causes of schizophrenia among family members: A community-based survey in Bali. *Psychiatric Services, 57*: 1795–1799.

Lamster, F., Kiener, J., Wagner, K., Rief, W., Görge, S. C., Iwaniuk, S., Leube, D., Falkenberg, I., Kluge, I., Kircher, T., & Mehl, S. (2018). Ist Wahn indirekt veränderbar? Ein stimmungsverbesserndes Konzept der kognitive Verhaltenstherapie für die stationäre Standardversorgung von Patienten mit schizophrenen Störungen = Are delusions indirectly alterable? A mood-stabilizing CBT-p concept for inpatients with schizophrenia. *Verhaltenstherapie, 28*: 138–146.

Landes, R. (1938). The abnormal among the Ojibwa Indians. *Journal of Abnormal and Social Psychology, 33*: 14–33.

Landy, D. (1985). Pibloktoq (hysteria) and Inuit nutrition: Possible implication of hypervitaminosis A. *Social Science & Medicine, 21*: 173–185.

Lanktree, M. B., Johansen, C. T., Joy, T. R., & Hegele, R. A. (2010). A translational view of the genetics of lipodystrophy and ectopic fat deposition. In: C. Bouchard (Ed.), *Progress in Molecular Biology and Translational Science* (pp. 159–196). San Diego, CA: Academic Press.

Laskemoen, J. F., Büchmann, C., Barrett, E. A., Collier-Høegh, M., Haatveit, B., Vedal, T. J., Ueland, T., Melle, I., Aas, M., & Simonsen, C. (2020). Do sleep disturbances contribute to cognitive impairments in schizophrenia spectrum and bipolar disorders? *European Archives of Psychiatry and Clinical Neuroscience, 270*: 749–759.

Laursen, T. M. (2019). Causes of premature mortality in schizophrenia: A review of literature published in 2018. *Current Opinion in Psychiatry, 32*: 388–393.

Laursen, T. M., Munk-Olsena, T., & Vestergaardb, M. (2012). Life expectancy and cardiovascular mortality in persons with schizophrenia. *Current Opinion in Psychiatry, 25*: 83–88.

Lawrence, R., Bradshaw, T., & Mairs, H. (2006). Group cognitive behavioural therapy for schizophrenia: A systematic review of the literature. *Journal of Psychiatric and Mental Health Nursing, 13*: 673–681.

Leão, T. S., Sundquist, J., Frank, G., Johansson, L.-M., Johansson, S.-E., & Sundquist, K. (2006). Incidence of schizophrenia or other psychoses in first- and second-generation immigrants: A national cohort study. *Journal of Nervous and Mental Disease, 194*: 27–33.

Lee, K. W., Woon, P. S., Teo, Y. Y., & Sim, K. (2012). Genome wide association studies (GWAS) and copy number variation (CNV) studies of the major psychoses: What have we learnt? *Neuroscience & Biobehavioral Reviews, 36*: 556–571.

Lee, Y., & Hu, P.-C. (1993). The effect of Chinese Qi-gong exercises and therapy on diseases and health. *Journal of Indian Psychology, 11*: 9–18.

Lehtinen, V., Aaltonen, J., Koffert, T., Räkköläinen, V., & Syvälahti, E. (2000). Two-year outcome in first-episode psychosis treated according to an integrated model. Is immediate neuroleptisation always needed? *European Psychiatry: The Journal of the Association of European Psychiatrists, 15*: 312–320.

Lehtonen, J. (2003). The dream between neuroscience and psychoanalysis: Has feeding an infant an impact on brain function and the capacity to create dream images in infants? *Psychoanalysis in Europe, 57*: 175–182.

Lehtonen, J., Könönen, M., Purhonen, M., Partanen, J., & Saarikoski, S. (2002). The effects of feeding on the electroencephalogram in 3- and 6-month-old infants. *Psychophysiology, 39*: 73–79.

Leonhardt, B. L., Hamm, J. A., Belanger, E. A., & Lysaker, P. H. (2015). Childhood sexual abuse moderates the relationship of self-reflectivity with increased emotional distress in schizophrenia. *Psychosis: Psychological, Social and Integrative Approaches, 7*: 195–205.

Lester, D. (2007). Suicide mortality in schizophrenics. In: R. Tatarelli, M. Pompili, & P. Girardi (Eds.), *Suicide in Schizophrenia* (pp. 19–29). New York: Nova Biomedical.

Leucht, S., Burkard, T., Henderson, J., Maj, M., & Sartorius, N. (2007). Physical illness and schizophrenia: A review of the literature. *Acta Psychiatrica Scandinavica, 116*: 317–333.

Leuzinger-Bohleber, M. (2016). Enactments in transference: Embodiment, trauma and depression. What have psychoanalysis and the neurosciences to offer to each other? In: S. Weigel & G. Scharbert (Eds.), *A Neuro-Psychoanalytical Dialogue for Bridging Freud and the Neurosciences* (pp. 33–46). Cham, Switzerland: Springer International.

Levin, F. M. (2011). *Psyche and Brain: The Biology of Talking Cures*. New York: Routledge.

Lewis, S., & Lieberman, J. (2008). CATIE and CutLASS: Can we handle the truth? *British Journal of Psychiatry, 192*: 161–163.

Lewis-Fernáandez, R. (1996). Cultural formulation of psychiatric diagnosis: Case No. 02 Diagnosis and treatment of *Nervios* and *Ataques* in a female Puerto Rican migrant. *Culture, Medicine, and Psychiatry: An International Journal of Cross-Cultural Health Research, 20*: 155–163.

Lidz, T., & Fleck, S. (1960). Schizophrenia, human integration, and the role of the family. In: D. D. Jackson (Ed.), *The Etiology of Schizophrenia* (pp. 323–345). Oxford: Basic Books.

Lieberman, F. (1984). Singular and plural objects: Thoughts on object relations theory. *Child & Adolescent Social Work Journal, 1*: 153–167.

Lieberman, J. A., Stroup, T. S., McEvoy, J. P., Swartz, M. S., Rosenheck, R. A., Perkins, D. O., Keefe, R. S. E., Davis, S. M., Lebowitz, B. D., Severe, J., & Hsiao, J. K. (2005). Effectiveness of antipsychotic drugs in patients with chronic schizophrenia. *New England Journal of Medicine, 353*: 1209–1223.

Lim, R. F., & Lin, K.-M. (1996). Cultural formulation of psychiatric diagnosis: Case No. 03: Psychosis following Qi-Gong in a Chinese immigrant. *Culture, Medicine and Psychiatry, 20*: 369–378.

Lindberg, J. (1974). American Eye: Wendigo: A fiction, a fantasy. *North American Review, 259*: 8–11.

Loewald, H. (1960). On the therapeutic action of psychoanalysis. *International Journal of Psychoanalysis, 41*: 16–33.

London, N. J. (1973a). An essay on psychoanalytic theory: Two theories of schizophrenia: I. Review and critical assessment of the development of the two theories. *International Journal of Psychoanalysis, 54*: 169–178.

London, N. J. (1973b). An essay on psychoanalytic theory: Two theories of schizophrenia: II. Discussion and restatement of the specific theory of schizophrenia. *International Journal of Psychoanalysis, 54*: 179–193.

López-Muñoz, F., Alamo, C., Cuenca, E., Shen, W. W., Clervoy, P., & Rubio, G. (2005). History of the discovery and clinical introduction of chlorpromazine. *Annals of Clinical Psychiatry, 17*: 113–135.

Lorenzo, C. V., Baca-Garcia, E., Diaz-Hernandez, M., Botillo-Martin, C., Perez-Rodriguez, M. M., Fernandez-Ramos, C., Saiz-Gonzalez, M. D., Quintero-Gutierrez, F. J., Saiz-Ruiz, J., Piqueras, J. F., de Rivera, J. L. G., & de Leon, J. (2006). Association between the T102C polymorphism of the serotonin-2A receptor gene and schizophrenia. *Progress in Neuro-Psychopharmacology & Biological Psychiatry, 30*: 1136–1138.

Lublin, H., & Eberhard, J. (2008). Content versus delivery: Challenges and options in the treatment of schizophrenia. *European Neuropsychopharmacology, 18*: v–vi.

Lucas, R. (2003). The relationship between psychoanalysis and schizophrenia. *International Journal of Psychoanalysis, 84*: 3–9.

Luhrmann, T. M. (2007). Social defeat and the culture of chronicity: Or, why schizophrenia does so well over there and so badly here. *Culture, Medicine, and Psychiatry: An International Journal of Cross-Cultural Health Research, 31*: 135–172.

Lysaker, P. H., Beattie, N. L., Strasburger, A. M., & Davis, L. W. (2005). Reported history of child sexual abuse in schizophrenia: Associations with heightened symptom levels and poorer participation over four months in vocational rehabilitation. *Journal of Nervous and Mental Disease, 193*: 790–795.

Lysaker, P. H., Meyer, P. S., Evans, J. D., Clements, C. A., & Marks, K. A. (2001). Childhood sexual trauma and psychosocial functioning in adults with schizophrenia. *Psychiatric Services, 52*: 1485–1488.

Lysaker, P. H., Nees, M. A., Lancaster, R. S., & Davis, L. W. (2004). Vocational function among persons with schizophrenia with and without history of childhood sexual trauma. *Journal of Traumatic Stress, 17*: 435–438.

Mahler, M. S. (1952). On child psychosis and schizophrenia: Autistic and symbiotic infantile psychoses. *Psychoanalytic Study of the Child, 7*: 286–305.

Mahler, M. S., & Furer, M. (1968). *On Human Symbiosis and the Vicissitudes of Individuation: I. Infantile Psychosis.* Oxford: International Universities Press.

Marini, S., Di Tizio, L., Dezi, S., Armuzzi, S., Pelaccia, S., Valchera, A., Sepede, G., Girinelli, G., De Berardis, D., Martinotti, G., Gambi, F., & Di Giannantonio, M. (2016). The bridge between two worlds: Psychoanalysis and fMRI. *Reviews in the Neurosciences, 27*: 219–229.

Marneros, A. (2007). Do schizoaffective disorders exist at all? *Acta Psychiatrica Scandinavica, 115*: 162.

Masciotra, L., Landreau, F., Conesa, H. A., & Erausquin, G. A. de. (2005). Pathophysiology of schizophrenia: A new look at the role of dopamine. In: M. V. Lang (Ed.), *Trends in Schizophrenia Research* (pp. 27–44). Hauppauge, NY: Nova Biomedical.

Mateen, B. A., Hill, C. S., Biddie, S. C., & Menon, D. K. (2017). DNA methylation: Basic biology and application to traumatic brain injury. *Journal of Neurotrauma, 34*: 2379–2388.

Maurel, M., Belzeaux, R., Adida, M., Fakra, E., Cermolacce, M., Da Fonseca, D., & Azorin, J.-M. (2011). Schizophrénie, cognition et psycho-éducation = Schizophrenia, cognition and psychoeducation. *L'Encéphale: Revue de Psychiatrie Clinique Biologique et Thérapeutique, 37*(Suppl 2): S151–S154.

Mausbach, B. T., Bucardo, J., McKibbin, C. L., Goldman, S. R., Jeste, D. V., Patterson, T. L., Cardenas, V., & Barrio, C. (2008). Evaluation of a culturally tailored skills intervention for Latinos with persistent psychotic disorders. *American Journal of Psychiatric Rehabilitation, 11*: 61–75.

May, P. (1968). *Treatment of Schizophrenia; A Comparative Study of Five Treatment Methods.* Santa Rosa, CA: Science House.

McCarroll, S. A., & Altshuler, D. M. (2007). Copy-number variation and association studies of human disease. *Nature Genetics, 39*: S37–S42.

McDougall, J. (1986). *Theatres of the Mind: Illusion and Truth on the Psychoanalytic Stage.* London: Free Association.

McGee, H. F. (1972). Windigo psychosis. *American Anthropologist, 74*: 244–246.

McGrath, J. J. (2006). Variations in the incidence of schizophrenia: Data versus dogma. *Schizophrenia Bulletin, 32*: 195–197.

McGrath, J. J., Brown, A., & St Clair, D. (2011). Prevention and schizophrenia—the role of dietary factors. *Schizophrenia Bulletin, 37*: 272–283.

Menninger, K. (1919a). Psychoses associated with influenza: I. General data: Statistical analysis. *Journal of the American Medical Association, 72*: 235–241.

Menninger, K. (1919b). Psychoses associated with influenza: II. Specific data. An expository analysis. *Archives of Neurology & Psychiatry, 2*: 291–337.

Menninger, K. (1920). Influenza psychoses in successive epidemics. *Archives of Neurology & Psychiatry, 3*: 57–60.

Menninger, K. (1922). Reversible schizophrenia. *American Journal of Psychiatry, 78*: 573–588.

Menninger, K. (1926). Influenza and schizophrenia. An analysis of post-influenzal "dementia precox," as of 1918, and five years later further studies of the psychiatric aspects of influenza. *American Journal of Psychiatry, 151*: 182–187.

Menninger, K. (1928). The schizophrenic syndrome as a product of acute infectious disease. *Archives of Neurology & Psychiatry, 20*: 464–481.

Meyer, U., Feldon, J., Schedlowski, M., & Yee, B. K. (2006). Immunological stress at the maternal-foetal interface: A link between neurodevelopment and adult psychopathology. *Brain, Behavior, and Immunity, 20*: 378–388.

Meyer, U., Murray, P. J., Unwyler, A., Yee, B. K., Schedlowski, M., & Feldon J. (2008). Adult behavioral and pharmacological dysfunctions following disruption of the fetal brain balance between pro-inflammatory and IL-10-mediated anti-inflammatory signaling. *Molecular Psychiatry, 13*: 208–221.

Meyer, U., Nyffeler, M., Knuesel, I., Yee, B. K., & Feldon, J. (2008). Relative prenatal and postnatal maternal contributions to schizophrenia-related neurochemical dysfunction after in utero immune challenge. *Neuropsychopharmacology, 33*: 441–446.

Miller, B. J., Buckley, P., Seabolt, W., Mellor, A., & Kirkpatrick, B. (2011). Meta-analysis of cytokine alterations in schizophrenia: Clinical status and antipsychotic effects. *Biological Psychiatry, 70*: 663–671.

Miller, M. J. (2011). *Ancestral Indigenous Culture and Historical-Transgenerational Trauma: Rethinking Schizophrenia in African Americans*. Ann Arbor, MI: ProQuest Information & Learning.

Miller, P., Lawrie, S. M., Hodges, A., Clafferty, R., Cosway, R., & Johnstone, E. C. (2001). Genetic liability, illicit drug use, life stress and psychotic symptoms: Preliminary findings from the Edinburgh study of people at high risk for schizophrenia. *Social Psychiatry and Psychiatric Epidemiology, 36*: 338–342.

Mishra, A., Mishra, A. K., & Jha, S. (2018). Effect of traditional medicine brahmi vati and bacoside A-rich fraction of Bacopa monnieri on acute pentylene-tetrzole-induced seizures, amphetamine-induced model of schizophrenia, and scopolamine-induced memory loss in laboratory animals. *Epilepsy & Behavior, 80*: 144–151.

Mitsadali, I., Grayson, B., Idris, N. F., Watson, L., Burgess, M., & Neill, J. (2020). Aerobic exercise improves memory and prevents cognitive deficits of relevance to schizophrenia in an animal model. *Journal of Psychopharmacology, 34*: 695–708.

Mittal, V. A., Saczawa, M. E., Walker, E., Willhite, R., & Walder, D. (2008). Prenatal exposure to viral infection and conversion among adolescents at high-risk for psychotic disorders. *Schizophrenia research, 99*: 375–376.

Modell, A. H. (1981). Does metapsychology still exist? *International Journal of Psychoanalysis, 62*: 391–402.

Møllerhøj, J., Os Stølan, L., Erdner, A., Hedberg, B., Stahl, K., Riise, J., Jedenius, E., & Rise, M. B. (2019). "I live, I don't work, but I live a very normal life"—A qualitative interview study of Scandinavian user experiences of schizophrenia, antipsychotic medication, and personal recovery processes. *Perspectives in Psychiatric Care, 56*: 371–378.

Moore, L. D., Le, T., & Fan, G. (2013). DNA methylation and its basic function. *Neuropsychopharmacology, 38*: 23–38.

Moran, E. K, Gold, J. M., Carter, C. S., MacDonald, A. W., & Ragland, J. D. (2020). Both unmedicated and medicated individuals with schizophrenia show impairments across a wide array of cognitive and reinforcement learning tasks. *Psychological Medicine* (August 17): 1–11.

Moreno, J. L., Kurita, M., Holloway, T., López, J., Cadagan, R., Martínez-Sobrido, L., García-Sastre, A., & González-Maeso, J. (2011). Maternal influenza viral infection causes schizophrenia- like alterations of 5-HT2A and mGlu$_2$ receptors in the adult offspring. *Journal of Neuroscience, 31*: 1863–1872.

Mueser, K. T., & Berenbaum, H. (1990). Psychodynamic treatment of schizophrenia: Is there a future? *Psychological Medicine, 20*: 253–262.

Mulder, M. B. (2009). Serial monogamy as polygyny or polyandry? Marriage in the Tanzanian Pimbwe. *Human Nature, 20*: 130–150.

Mulle, J. G. (2012). Schizophrenia genetics: Progress, at last. *Current Opinion in Genetics & Development, 22*: 238–244.

Mullen, P. E. (2005). Child sexual abuse and schizophrenia: Author's reply. *British Journal of Psychiatry, 186*: 76.

Murray, R. M., Grech, A., Phillips, P., & Johnson, S. (2003). What is the relationship between substance abuse and schizophrenia? In:

R. M. Murray, P. B. Jones, E. Susser, J. van Os, & M. Cannon (Eds.), *The Epidemiology of Schizophrenia* (pp. 317–342). Cambridge: Cambridge University Press.

Nelson, C. L. M., Amsbaugh, H. M., Reilly, J. L., Rosen, C., Marvin, R. W., Ragozzino, M. E., Bishop, J. R., Sweeney, J. A., & Hill, S. K. (2018). Beneficial and adverse effects of antipsychotic medication on cognitive flexibility are related to COMT genotype in first episode psychosis. *Schizophrenia Research, 202*: 212–216.

Ng, B.-Y. (1999). Qigong-induced mental disorders: A review. *Australian and New Zealand Journal of Psychiatry, 33*: 197–206.

Niebuhr, D. W., Millikan, A. M., Cowan, D. N., Yolken, R., Li, Y., & Weber, N. S. (2008). Selected infectious agents and risk of schizophrenia among U.S. military personnel. *American Journal of Psychiatry, 165*: 99–106.

Niehaus, D., Oosthuizen, P., Lochner, C., Emsley, R. A., Jordaan, E., Mbanga, N. I., Keyter, N., Laurent, C., Deleuze, J.-F., & Stein, D. J. (2004). A culture-bound syndrome "Amafufunyana" and a culture-specific event "Ukuthwasa": Differentiated by a family history of schizophrenia and other psychiatric disorders. *Psychopathology, 37*: 59–63.

Nightingale, L. C., & McQueeney, D. A. (1996). Group therapy for schizophrenia: Combining and expanding the psychoeducational model with supportive psychotherapy. *International Journal of Group Psychotherapy, 46*: 517–533.

Nixon, N. L., & Doody, G. A. (2005). Official psychiatric morbidity and the incidence of schizophrenia 1881–1994. *Psychological Medicine, 35*: 1145–1153.

Noack, F., & Calegari, F. (2014). Micro-RNAs meet epigenetics to make for better brains. *EMBO Reports, 15*: 1224–1225.

Novick, J., & Kelly, K. (1970). Projection and externalization. *Psychoanalytic Study of the Child, 25*: 69–95.

Ødegård, Ø. (1932). *Emigration and Insanity—A Study of Mental Disease among the Norwegian Born Population of Minnesota.* Copenhagen: Levin & Munksgaard.

Ohara, K. (2007). The n-3 polyunsaturated fatty acid/dopamine hypothesis of schizophrenia. *Progress in Neuro-Psychopharmacology & Biological Psychiatry, 31*: 469–474.

Olinick, S. L. (1980). *The Psychotherapeutic Instrument.* New York: Jason Aronson.

Opler, M. K. (1959). *Culture and Mental Health—Cross-Cultural Studies.* New York: Macmillan.

Ortiz-Medina, M. B., Perea, M., Torales, J., Ventriglio, A., Vitrani, G., Aguilar, L., & Roncero, C. (2018). Cannabis consumption and psychosis or schizophrenia development. *International Journal of Social Psychiatry, 64*: 690–704.

Ottet, M.-C., Schaer, M., Cammoun, L., Schneider, M., Debbané, M., Thiran, J.-P., & Eliez, S. (2013). Reduced fronto-temporal and limbic connectivity in the 22q112 deletion syndrome: Vulnerability markers for developing schizophrenia? *PLoS ONE, 8*: e58429.

Pandurangi, A. K., & Buckley, P. F. (2020). Inflammation, antipsychotic drugs, and evidence for effectiveness of anti-inflammatory agents in schizophrenia. In: G. M. Khandaker, U. Meyer, & P. B. Jones (Eds.), *Neuroinflammation and Schizophrenia* (pp. 227–244). Cham, Switzerland: Springer International.

Pang, N., Thrichelvam, N., & Naing, K. O. (2017). Olanzapine-induced pancytopenia: A rare but worrying complication. *East Asian Archives of Psychiatry, 27*: 35–37.

Pao, P.-N. (1979). *Schizophrenic Disorders: Theory and Treatment from a Psychodynamic Point of View.* New York: International Universities Press.

Pardiñas, A. F., Holmans, P., Pocklington, A. J., Escott-Price, V., Ripke, S., Carrera, N., ... (140 more) & Walters, J. T. R. (2018). Common schizophrenia alleles are enriched in mutation-intolerant genes and in regions under strong background selection. *Nature Genetics, 50*: 381–389.

Parle, J. (2003). Witchcraft or madness? The Amandiki of Zululand, 1894–1914. *Journal of Southern African Studies, 29*: 105–132.

Peltzer, K. (1999). Faith healing for mental and social disorders in the northern province [South Africa]. *Journal of Religion in Africa, 29*: 387–402.

Potvin, S., Stip, E., Sepehry, A. A., Gendron, A., Bah, R., & Kouassi, E. (2008). Inflammatory cytokine alterations in schizophrenia: A systematic quantitative review. *Biological Psychiatry, 63*: 801–808.

Poulet, E., Brunelin, J., Kallel, L., D'Amato, T., & Saoud, M. (2008). Maintenance treatment with transcranial magnetic stimulation in a patient with late-onset schizophrenia. *American Journal of Psychiatry, 165*: 537–538.

Prasad, K. M. R., Shirts, B. H., Yolken, R. H., Jeshava, M. S., & Nimgaonkar, V. L. (2007a). Brain morphological changes associated with exposure to HSV1 in first-episode schizophrenia. *Molecular Psychiatry, 12*: 105–113.

Prasad, K. M. R., Shirts, B. H., Yolken, R. H., Jeshava, M. S., & Nimgaonkar, V. L. (2007b). HSV1 exposure affects prefrontal cortical structure in schizophrenia patients. *Molecular Psychiatry, 12*: 1.

Pratt, L. A. (2012). Characteristics of adults with serious mental illness in the United States household population in 2007. *Psychiatric Services, 63*: 1042–1046.

Ptak, S. E., & Lachmann, M. (2003). On the evolution of polygyny: A theoretical examination of the polygyny threshold model. *Behavioral Ecology, 14*: 201–211.

Purhonen, M., Pääkkönen, A., Yppärilä, H., Lehtonen, J., & Karhu, J. (2001). Dynamic behavior of the auditory N100 elicited by a baby's cry. *International Journal of Psychophysiology, 41*: 271–278.

Rado, J. T., & Hernandez, E. I. (2014). Therapeutic neuromodulation for treatment of schizophrenia. In: P. G. Janicak, S. R. Marder, R. Tandon, & M. Goldman (Eds.), *Schizophrenia: Recent Advances in Diagnosis and Treatment* (pp. 139–160). New York: Springer Science.

Rakitzi, S., Georgila, P., & Becker-Woitag, A. P. (2020). The recovery process for individuals with schizophrenia in the context of evidence-based psycho-therapy and rehabilitation: A systematic review. *European Psychologist, 26*: 96–111.

Ramamourty, P., Menon, V., & Aparna, M. (2014). Koro presenting as acute and transient psychosis: Implications for classification. *Asian Journal of Psychiatry, 10*: 116–117.

Ran, M.-S., Chen, E. Y.-H., Conwell, Y., Lai-Wan Chan, C., Yip, P. S. F., Xiang, M.-Z., & Caine, E. D. (2007). Mortality in people with schizophrenia in rural China: 10-year cohort study. *British Journal of Psychiatry, 190*: 237–242.

Rapaport, D. (1951). *Organization and Pathology of Thought: Selected Sources.* New York: Columbia University Press.

Rashno, M. M., Fallahi, S., Arab-Mazar, Z., & Dana, H. (2019). Seromolecular assess of Toxoplasma gondii infection in pregnant women and neonatal umbilical cord blood. *EXCLI Journal, 18*: 1–7.

Rathbone, J., Zhang, L., Zhang, M., Xia, J., Liu, X., Yang, Y., & Adams, C. E. (2007). Chinese herbal medicine for schizophrenia: Cochrane systematic review of randomised trials. *British Journal of Psychiatry, 190*: 379–384.

Read, J., Agar, K., Argyle, N., & Aderhold, V. (2003). Sexual and physical abuse during childhood and adulthood as predictors of hallucinations, delusions and thought disorder. *Psychology and Psychotherapy: Theory, Research and Practice, 76*: 1–22.

Read, J., van Os, J., Morrison, A. P., & Ross, C. A. (2005). Childhood trauma, psychosis and schizophrenia: A literature review with theoretical and clinical implications. *Acta Psychiatrica Scandinavica, 112*: 330–350.

Richard, M. D., & Brahm, N. C. (2012). Schizophrenia and the immune system: Pathophysiology, prevention, and treatment. *American Journal of Health-System Pharmacy, 69*: 757–766.

Richetto, J., & Meyer, U. (2020). Epigenetic modifications in schizophrenia and related disorders: Molecular scars of environmental exposures and source of phenotypic variability. *Biological Psychiatry, 89*: 215–226.

Robinson, D. S. (2008). Mortality risks and antipsychotics. *Primary Psychiatry, 15*: 21–23.

Roffman, J. L., Marci, C. D., Glick, D. M., Dougherty, D. D., & Rauch, S. L. (2005). Neuroimaging and the functional neuroanatomy of psychotherapy. *Psychological Medicine, 35*: 1385–1398.

Rogers, J. P., Chesney, E., Oliver, D., Pollak, T. A., McGuire, P., Fusar-Poli, P., Zandi, M. S., Lewis, G., & David, A. S. (2020). Psychiatric and neuro-psychiatric presentations associated with severe coronavirus infections: A systematic review and meta-analysis with comparison to the COVID-19 pandemic. *Lancet Psychiatry, 7*: 611–627.

Rohrl, V. J. (1970). A nutritional factor in Windigo psychosis. *American Anthropologist, 72*: 97–101.

Rokita, K. I., Dauvermann, M. R., Mothersill, D., Holleran, L., Holland, J., Costello, L., Cullen, C., Kane, R., McKernan, D., Morris, D. W., Kelly, J., Gill, M., Corvin, A., Hallahan, B., McDonald, C., & Donohoe, G. (2020). Childhood trauma, parental bonding, and social cognition in patients with schizophrenia and healthy adults. *Journal of Clinical Psychology, 77*: 241–253.

Rosenfeld, D. (1992). *The Psychotic: Aspects of the Personality*. New York: Routledge.

Rosenfeld, H. A. (1965). *Psychotic States: A Psycho-analytical Approach*. London: Hogarth.

Roser, P. (2019). Cannabis und schizophrenie—Risikofaktoren, diagnostische einordnung und auswirkungen auf verlauf und prognose. *Forensische Psychiatrie, Psychologie, Kriminologie, 13*: 225–232.

Ross, C. A. (2006). Dissociation and psychosis: The need for integration of theory and practice. In: J. O. Johannessen, B. V. Martindale, & J. Cullberg (Eds.), *Evolving Psychosis* (pp. 238–254). New York: Routledge/Taylor & Francis.

Ross, C. A. (2014). Dissociation in classical texts on schizophrenia. *Psychosis: Psychological, Social and Integrative Approaches, 6*: 342–354.

Rossello, J.-J., Gaillard, G., & Neuilly, M.-T. (2013). Une institution en quête de limites. Le mythe de Tom Sawyer: Un objet transitionnel collectif. *Revue de Psychothérapie Psychanalytique de Groupe, 60*: 141–152.

Rumbaugh, G., & Miller, C. A. (2011). Epigenetic changes in the brain: Measuring global histone modifications. *Methods in Molecular Biology, 670*: 263–274.

Ryan, J. E., Veliz, P., McCabe, S. E., Stoddard, S. A., & Boyd, C. J. (2020). Association of early onset of cannabis, cigarette, other drug use and schizophrenia or psychosis. *Schizophrenia Research, 215*: 482–484.

Sabe, M., Kaiser, S., & Sentissi, O. (2020). Physical exercise for negative symptoms of schizophrenia: Systematic review of randomized controlled trials and meta-analysis. *General Hospital Psychiatry, 62*: 13–20.

Saha, S., Chant, D., & McGrath, J. (2007). A systematic review of mortality in schizophrenia: Is the differential mortality gap worsening over time? *Archives of General Psychiatry, 64*: 1123–1131.

Saha, S., Chant, D. C., Welham, J. L., & McGrath, J. J. (2006). The incidence and prevalence of schizophrenia varies with latitude. *Acta Psychiatrica Scandinavica, 114*: 36–39.

Saha, S., Welham, J., Chant, D., & McGrath, J. (2006). Incidence of schizophrenia does not vary with economic status of the country: Evidence from a systematic review. *Social Psychiatry and Psychiatric Epidemiology, 41*: 338–340.

Salone, A., Di Giacinto, A., Lai, C., De Berardis, D., Iasevoli, F., Fornaro, M., De Risio, L., Santacroce, R., Martinotti, G., & Giannantonio, M. D. (2016). The interface between neuroscience and neuro-psychoanalysis: Focus on brain connectivity. *Frontiers in Human Neuroscience, 10*: 20.

Sanderson, I. T. (1963). Some preliminary notes on traditions of submen in arctic and subarctic North America. *Genus, 19*: 145–162.

Sandler, J., & Joffe, W. G. (1969). Towards a basic psychoanalytic model. *International Journal of Psychoanalysis, 50*: 79–90.

Saravanan, B., Jacob, K. S., Johnson, S., Prince, M., Bhugra, D., & David, A. S. (2007a). Assessing insight in schizophrenia: East meets West. *British Journal of Psychiatry, 190*: 243–247.

Saravanan, B., Jacob, K. S., Johnson, S., Prince, M., Bhugra, D., & David, A. S. (2007b). Belief models in first episode schizophrenia in South India. *Social Psychiatry and Psychiatric Epidemiology: The International Journal for Research in Social and Genetic Epidemiology and Mental Health Services, 42*: 446–451.

Sarter, M., Nelson, C. L., & Bruno, J. P. (2005). Cortical cholinergic transmission and cortical information processing in schizophrenia. *Schizophrenia Bulletin, 31*: 117–138.

Saxe, R. (2015, December). Why I captured this MRI of a mother and child. *Smithsonian Magazine.*

Schore, A. N. (2015). *Affect Regulation and the Origin of the Self: The Neurobiology of Emotional Development.* New York: Routledge.

Schulmann, G. (2004). Psychotherapy of schizophrenia and projective identification. Presented at the International Psychoanalytic Association Meeting, New Orleans, LA.

Schulz, C. G. (1983). Technique with schizophrenic patients. *Psychoanalytic Inquiry, 3*: 105–124.

Schürhoff, F., Laguerre, A., Fisher, H., Etain, B., Méary, A., Soussy, C., Szöke, A., & Leboyer, M. (2009). Self-reported childhood trauma correlates with schizotypal measures in schizophrenia but not bipolar pedigrees. *Psychological Medicine, 39*: 365–370.

Schwab, S. G., & Wildenauer, D. B. (2008). Research on causes for schizophrenia: Are we close? *Schizophrenia Research, 102*: 29–30.

Scull, A. (2005). *Madhouse: A Tragic Tale of Megalomania and Modern Medicine.* New Haven, CT: Yale University Press.

Searles, H. F. (1959). Integration and differentiation in schizophrenia. *British Journal of Medical Psychology, 32*: 261–281.

Searles, H. F. (1961). Phases of patient-therapist interaction in the psychotherapy of chronic schizophrenia. *British Journal of Medical Psychology, 34*: 169–193.

Searles, H. F. (1979). *Countertransference and Related Subjects: Selected Papers.* Madison, CT: International Universities Press.

Searles, H. F. (1986). *Collected Papers on Schizophrenia and Related Subjects.* London: Routledge.

Seeman, P. (2000). Antipsychotic drugs, dopamine D2 receptors, and schizophrenia. In: M. S. Lidow (Ed.), *Neurotransmitter Receptors in Actions of Antipsychotic Medications* (pp. 43–63). Boca Raton, FL: CRC.

Segal, H. (1988). *Introduction to the Work of Melanie Klein.* London: Routledge.

Sells, J. (2000). *Unante.* Hollywood, CA: W. M. Hawley.

Sepehry, A. A., Potvin, S., Élie, R., & Stip, E. (2007). Selective serotonin reuptake inhibitor (SSRI) add-on therapy for the negative symptoms of schizophrenia: A meta-analysis. *Journal of Clinical Psychiatry, 68*: 604–610.

Setién-Suero, E., Neergaard, K., Ortiz-García de la Foz, V., Suárez-Pinilla, P., Martínez-García, O., Crespo-Facorro, B., & Ayesa-Arriola, R. (2019). Stopping cannabis use benefits outcome in psychosis: Findings from 10-year follow-up study in the PAFIP-cohort. *Acta Psychiatrica Scandinavica, 140*: 349–359.

Severance, E. G., Prandovszky, E., Castiglione, J., & Yolken, R. H. (2015). Gastroenterology issues in schizophrenia: Why the gut matters. *Current Psychiatry Reports, 17*: 27.

Severance, E. G., & Yolken, R. H. (2020). From infection to the microbiome: An evolving role of microbes in schizophrenia. *Current Topics in Behavioral Neurosciences, 44*: 67–84.

Severance, E. G., Yolken, R. H., & Eaton, W. W. (2016). Autoimmune diseases, gastrointestinal disorders and the microbiome in schizophrenia: More than a gut feeling. *Schizophrenia Research, 176*: 23–35.

Shao, X., Lv, N., Liao, J., Long, J., Xue, R., Ai, N., Xu, D., & Fan, X. (2019). Copy number variation is highly correlated with differential gene expression: A pan-cancer study. *BMC Medical Genetics, 20*: 175.

Shonin, E., Van Gordon, W., & Griffiths, M. D. (2014). Cognitive behavioral therapy (CBT) and meditation awareness training (MAT) for the treatment of co-occurring schizophrenia and pathological gambling: A case study. *International Journal of Mental Health and Addiction, 12*: 181–196.

Shekunov, J. (2016). Immigration and risk of psychiatric disorders: A review of existing literature. *American Journal of Psychiatry Residents' Journal, 11*: 3–5.

Shimada, T., Ito, S., Makabe, A., Yamanushi, A., Takenaka, A., & Kobayashi, M. (2019). Aerobic exercise and cognitive functioning in schizophrenia: A pilot randomized controlled trial. *Psychiatry Research, 282*:112638.

Silva, M. A., & Restrepo, D. (2019). Recuperación funcional en la esquizofrenia = Functional recovery in schizophrenia. *Revista Colombiana de Psiquiatría, 48*: 252–260.

Sim, K., Chan, Y. H., Chua, T. H., Mahendran, R., Chong, S. A., & McGorry, P. (2006). Physical comorbidity, insight, quality of life and global functioning in first episode schizophrenia: A 24-month, longitudinal outcome study. *Schizophrenia Research, 88*: 82–89.

Sim, K., Chua, T. H., Chan, Y. H., Mahendran, R., & Chong, S. A. (2006). Psychiatric comorbidity in first episode schizophrenia: A 2 year, longitudinal outcome study. *Journal of Psychiatric Research, 40*: 656–663.

Simeone, J. C., Ward, A. J., Rotella, P., Collins, J., & Windisch, R. (2015). An evaluation of variation in published estimates of schizophrenia prevalence from 1990–2013: A systematic literature review. *BMC Psychiatry, 15*: 1–14.

Simpson, M. A. (1995). Gullible's travels, or the importance of being multiple. In: L. M. Cohen, J. N. Berzoff, & M. R. Elin (Eds.), *Dissociative Identity Disorder: Theoretical and Treatment Controversies* (pp. 87–134). Northvale, NJ: Jason Aronson.

Singh, B., & Chaudhuri, T. K. (2014). Role of C-reactive protein in schizophrenia: An overview. *Psychiatry Research, 216*: 277–285.

Smigielski, L., Jagannath, V., Rössler, W., Walitza, S., & Grünblatt, E. (2020). Epigenetic mechanisms in schizophrenia and other psychotic disorders: A systematic review of empirical human findings. *Molecular Psychiatry, 25*: 1718–1748.

Sommer, I. E., de Witte, L., Begemann, M., & Kahn, R. S. (2012). Nonsteroidal anti-inflammatory drugs in schizophrenia: Ready for practice or a good start? A meta-analysis. *Journal of Clinical Psychiatry, 73*: 414–419.

Spanos, N. P., & Gottlieb, J. (1979). Demonic possession, Mesmerism, and hysteria: A social psychological perspective on their historical interrelations. *Journal of Abnormal Psychology, 88*: 527–546.

Spataro, J., Mullen, P. E., Burgess, P. M., Wells, D. L., & Moss, S. A. (2004). Impact of child sexual abuse on mental health: Prospective study in males and females. *British Journal of Psychiatry, 184*: 416–421.

Spitz, R. A. (1965). *The First Year of Life: A Psychoanalytic Study of Normal and Deviant Development of Object Relations.* Oxford: International Universities Press.

Staudt, M. D., Herring, E. Z., Gao, K., Miller, J. P., & Sweet, J. A. (2019). Evolution in the treatment of psychiatric disorders: From psychosurgery to psychopharmacology to neuromodulation. *Frontiers in Neuroscience, 13*: 108.

Steel, C. (Ed.) (2013). *CBT for Schizophrenia: Evidence-based Interventions and Future Directions.* Oxford: Wiley-Blackwell.

Stefansson, H., Meyer-Lindenberg, A., Steinberg, S., Magnusdottir, B., Morgen, K., Arnarsdottir, S., Bjornsdottir, G., Walters, G. B., Jonsdottir, G. A., Doyle, O. M., Tost, H., Grimm, O., Kristjansdottir, S., Snorrason, H., Davidsdottir, S. R., Gudmundsson, L. J., Jonsson, G. F., Stefansdottir, B., Helgadottir, I., Haraldsson, M., Jonsdottir, B., Thygesen, J. H., Schwarz, A. J., Didriksen, M., Stensbøl, T. B., Brammer, M., Kapur, S., Halldorsson, J. G., Hreidarsson, S., Saemundsen, E., Sigurdsson, E., & Stefansson, K. (2014). CNVs conferring risk of autism or schizophrenia affect cognition in controls. *Nature, 505*: 361–366.

Stern, D. N. (1985). *The Interpersonal World of the Infant: A View from Psychoanalysis and Developmental Psychology.* New York: Basic Books.

Stone, M. H. (1999). The history of the psychoanalytic treatment of schizophrenia. *Journal of the American Academy of Psychoanalysis, 27*: 583–601.

Sudak, D. M. (2004). Cognitive-behavioral therapy for schizophrenia. *Journal of Psychiatric Practice, 10*: 331–333.

Sullivan, H. S. (1962). *Schizophrenia as a Human Process.* New York: W. W. Norton.

Sullivan, P., Daly, M. J., & O'Donovan, M. (2012). Genetic architectures of psychiatric disorders: The emerging picture and its implications. *Nature Reviews Genetics, 13*: 537–551.

Sumiyoshi, T., Park, S., Jayathilake, K., Roy, A., Ertugrul, A., & Meltzer, H. Y. (2007). Effect of buspirone, a serotonin-sub(1A) partial agonist, on cognitive function in schizophrenia: A randomized, double-blind, placebo-controlled study. *Schizophrenia Research, 95*: 158–168.

Sutterland, A. L., Kuin, A., Kuiper, B., van Gool, T., Leboyer, M., Fond, G., & de Haan, L. (2019). Driving us mad: The association of Toxoplasma gondii with suicide attempts and traffic accidents—A systematic review and meta-analysis. *Psychological Medicine, 49*: 1608–1623.

Suvisaari, J. M., Haukka, J. K., Tanskanen, A. J., & Lönnqvist, J. K. (1999). Decline in the incidence of schizophrenia in Finnish cohorts born from 1954 to 1965. *Archives of General Psychiatry, 56*: 733–740.

Suwanlert, S. (1976). Neurotic and psychotic states attributed to Thai "Phii Pob" spirit possession. *Australian and New Zealand Journal of Psychiatry, 10*: 119–123.

Szumlinski, K. K., & Kippin, T. E. (2008). Homer: A genetic factor in schizophrenia? In: P. O'Donnell (Ed.), *Cortical Deficits in Schizophrenia: From Genes to Function* (pp. 29–72). New York: Springer Science.

Tähkä, V. (1993). *Mind and Its Treatment: A Psychoanalytic Approach*. Madison, CT: International Universities Press.

Tandon, R., Nasrallah, H. A., & Keshavan, M. S. (2010). Schizophrenia, "Just the Facts" 5. Treatment and prevention past, present, and future. *Schizophrenia Research, 122*: 1–23.

Taquet, M., Luciano, S., Geddes, J. R., & Harrison, P. J. (2021). Bidirectional associations between COVID-19 and psychiatric disorder: Retrospective cohort studies of 62,354 COVID-19 cases in the USA. *Lancet Psychiatry, 8*: 130–140.

Thomann, P. A., Wolf, R. C., Nolte, H. M., Hirjak, D., Hofer, S., Seidl, U., Depping, M. S., Stieltjes, B., Maier-Hein, K., Sambataro, F., & Wüstenberg, T. (2017). Neuromodulation in response to electroconvulsive therapy in schizophrenia and major depression. *Brain Stimulation, 10*: 637–644.

Thygesen, J. H., Presman, A., Harju-Seppänen, J., Irizar, H., Jones, R., Kuchenbaecker, K., Lin, K., Alizadeh, B. Z., Austin-Zimmerman, I., Bartels-Velthuis, A., Bhat, A., Bruggeman, R., Cahn, W., Calafato, S., Crespo-Facorro, B., de Haan, L., de Zwarte, S., Di Forti, M., Díez-Revuelta, Á., Hall, J., [...] Bramon, E. (2020). Genetic copy number variants, cognition and psychosis: a meta-analysis and a family study. *Molecular Psychiatry*, 10.1038/s41380-020-0820-7. Advance online publication.

Tidd, C. W. (1937). Increasing reality acceptance by a schizoid personality during analysis. *Bulletin of the Menninger Clinic, 1*: 176–183.

Tidd, C. W. (1938). A note on the treatment of schizophrenia. *Bulletin of the Menninger Clinic, 2*: 89–93.

Tochigi, M., Okazaki, Y., Kato, N., & Sasaki, T. (2004). What causes seasonality of birth in schizophrenia? *Neuroscience Research, 48*: 1–11.

Torrey, E. F., Bartko, J. J., & Yolken, R. H. (2012). Toxoplasma gondii and other risk factors for schizophrenia: An update. *Schizophrenia Bulletin, 38*: 642–647.

Torsti, M. (1998). On motherhood. *Scandinavian Psychoanalytic Review, 21*: 53–76.

Tropp, J. (2003). The python and the crying tree: Interpreting tales of environmental and colonial power in the Transkei. *International Journal of African Historical Studies, 36*: 511–532.

Trudeau, K. J., Burtner, J., Villapiano, A. J., Jones, M., Butler, S. F., & Joshi, K. (2018). Burden of schizophrenia or psychosis-related symptoms in adults undergoing substance abuse evaluation. *Journal of Nervous and Mental Disease, 206*: 528–536.

Tsapakis, E.-M., Guillin, O., & Murray, R. M. (2003). Does dopamine sensitization underlie the association between schizophrenia and drug abuse? *Current Opinion in Psychiatry, 16*: S45–S52.

Turkington, D., Dudley, R., Warman, D. M., & Beck, A. T. (2004). Cognitive-behavioral therapy for schizophrenia: A review. *Journal of Psychiatric Practice, 10*: 5–16.

Turkington, D., Kingdon, D., & Chadwick, P. (2003). Cognitive-behavioural therapy for schizophrenia: Filling the therapeutic vacuum. *British Journal of Psychiatry, 183*: 98–99.

Tustin, F. (2018). *Autistic Barriers in Neurotic Patients.* New York: Routledge.

Udina, M., Foulon, H., Valdés, M., Bhattacharyya, S., & Martín-Santos, R. (2013). Dhat syndrome: A systematic review. *Psychosomatics: Journal of Consultation and Liaison Psychiatry, 54*: 212–218.

Valon, P. (2020). Gisela Pankow (1914–1998): Towards a psychoanalytic treatment of the psychoses. *International Journal of Psychoanalysis, 101*: 169–185.

Varvin, S., & Rosenbaum, B. (2014). West-East differences in habits and ways of thinking: The influence on understanding and teaching psychoanalytic therapy. In: D. E. Scharff & S. Varvin (Eds.), *Psychoanalysis in China* (pp. 123–136). London: Karnac.

Vaucher, J., Keating, B. J., Lasserre, A. M., Gan, W., Lyall, D. M., Ward, J., Smith, D. J., Pell, J. P., Sattar, N., Paré, G., & Holmes, M. V. (2018). Cannabis use and risk of schizophrenia: A Mendelian randomization study. *Molecular Psychiatry, 23*: 1287–1292.

Verlingue, M. (1986). Haute-Volta et "Psychose Abidjan-Niger". *Psychologie Medicale, 18*: 93–96.

Vidal, S., & Huguelet, P. (2019). Thérapie cognitive basée sur le concept de rétablissement pour la schizophrénie: Un cas clinique. *Journal de Thérapie Comportementale et Cognitive, 29*: 57–66.

Vitebsky, P. (1993). *Dialogues with the Dead: The Discussion of Mortality among the Sora of Eastern India.* Cambridge: Cambridge University Press.

Vitebsky, P. (2017). *Living without the Dead: Loss and Redemption in a Jungle Cosmos.* Chicago, IL: University of Chicago Press.

Vogel, M., Meier, J., Grönke, S., Waage, M., Schneider, W., Freyberger, H. J., & Klauer, T. (2011). Differential effects of childhood abuse and neglect: Mediation by posttraumatic distress in neurotic disorder and negative symptoms in schizophrenia? *Psychiatry Research, 189*: 121–127.

Volavka, J., Laska, E., Baker, S., Meisner, M., Czobor, P., & Krivelevich, I. (1997). History of violent behaviour and schizophrenia in different cultures: Analyses based on the WHO study on Determinants of Outcome of Severe Mental Disorders. *British Journal of Psychiatry, 171*: 9–14.

Volkan, K. (1994). *Dancing Among the Maenads: The Psychology of Compulsive Drug Use.* Bern, Switzerland: Peter Lang.

Volkan, K. (2013). A psychoanalytic view of the Sangha: Group functioning in Mahayana and Tibetan Buddhism. *Asian Journal of Humanities and Social Studies, 1*: 47–54.

Volkan, K. (2020a). Delusional misidentification syndromes: Psychopathology and culture. *Journal of Health and Medical Sciences, 3*: 288–301.

Volkan, K. (2020b). Encounter with the demonic: Western, eastern, and object relations approaches. *Psychology, 11*: 1454–1470.

Volkan, K. (2021). Hoarding and animal hoarding: Psychodynamic and transitional aspects. *Psychodynamic Psychiatry, 49*: 24–47.

Volkan, V. D. (1964). The observation and topographic study of the changing ego states of a schizophrenic patient. *British Journal of Medical Psychology, 37*: 239–255.

Volkan, V. D. (1976). *Primitive Internalized Object Relations: A Clinical Study of Schizophrenic, Borderline, and Narcissistic Patients.* New York: International Universities Press.

Volkan, V. D. (1981). *Linking Objects and Linking Phenomena.* New York: International Universities Press.

Volkan, V. D. (1986). Suitable targets of externalization and schizophrenia. In: D. B. Feinsilver (Ed.), *Towards a Comprehensive Model for Schizophrenic Disorders: Psychoanalytic Essays in Memory of Ping-Nie Pao* (pp. 125–153). Hillsdale, NJ: Analytic Press.

Volkan, V. D. (1987). *Six Steps in the Treatment of Borderline Personality Organization.* Northvale, NJ: Jason Aronson.

Volkan, V. D. (1988). *The Need to Have Enemies and Allies: From Clinical Practice to International Relationships.* Lanham, MD: Jason Aronson.

Volkan, V. D. (1990). The psychoanalytic psychotherapy of schizophrenia. In: L. B. Boyer & P. L. Giovacchini (Eds.), *Master Clinicians on Treating the Regressed Patient* (pp. 245–270). Lanham, MD: Jason Aronson.

Volkan, V. D. (1994). Identification with the therapist's functions and ego-building in the treatment of schizophrenia. *British Journal of Psychiatry, 164*: 77–82.

Volkan, V. D. (1995). *The Infantile Psychotic Self and Its Fates: Understanding and Treating Schizophrenics and Other Difficult Patients.* Lanham, MD: Jason Aronson.

Volkan, V. D. (2004a). *Blind Trust: Large Groups and Their Leaders in Times of Crisis and Terror.* Charlottesville, VA: Pitchstone.

Volkan, V. D. (2004b). Actualized unconscious fantasies and "therapeutic play" in adults' analyses: Further study of these concepts. In: A. Laine (Ed.), *Power of Understanding: Essays in Honour of Veikko Tähkä* (pp. 119–141). London: Karnac.

Volkan, V. D. (2005). The cat people revisited. In: S. Akhtar and V. D. Volkan (Eds.), *Mental Zoo: Animals in the Human Mind and Its Pathology* (pp. 265–289). Madison, CT: International Universities Press.

Volkan, V. D. (2006). *Killing in the Name of Identity: A Study of Bloody Conflicts.* Charlottesville, VA: Pitchstone.

Volkan, V. D. (2010). *Psychoanalytic Technique Expanded: A Textbook on Psychoanalytic Treatment.* London: Oa.

Volkan, V. D. (2015a). *A Nazi Legacy: Depositing, Transgenerational Transmission, Dissociation, and Remembering Through Action.* London: Routledge.

Volkan, V. D. (2015b). *Would-be Wife Killer: A Clinical Study of Primitive Mental Functions, Actualised Unconscious Fantasies, Satellite States, and Developmental Steps.* London: Karnac.

Volkan, V. D. (2017). *Immigrants and Refugees: Trauma, Perennial Mourning, Prejudice, and Border Psychology.* London: Karnac.

Volkan, V. D. (2019). *A Study of Ghosts in the Human Psyche: Story of a Muslim Armenian.* Banbury, UK: Phoenix.

Volkan, V. D., (2020). *Large-Group Psychology: Racism, Societal Divisions, Narcissistic Leaders, and Who We Are Now.* Banbury, UK: Phoenix.

Volkan, V. D. (2021). *Sexual Addiction and Hunger for Maternal Care: Psychoanalytic Concepts and the Art of Supervision.* Banbury, UK: Phoenix.

Volkan, V. D., & Akhtar, S. (1979). The symptoms of schizophrenia: Contributions of the structural theory and object relations theory. In: L. Saretsky, G. D. Goldman, & D. S. Milman (Eds.), *Integrating Ego Psychology and Object Relations* (pp. 270–285). Dubuque, IA: Kendall/Hunt.

Volkan, V. D., & Akhtar, S. (Eds.) (1997). *The Seed of Madness: Constitution, Environment, and Fantasy in the Organization of the Psychotic Core*. Madison, CT: International Universities Press.

Volkan, V. D., & Ast, G. (1997). A room within a room: Clinical observations of a "mad" core. In: V. D. Volkan & S. Akhtar (Eds.), *The Seed of Madness: Constitution, Environment, and Fantasy in the Organization of the Psychotic Core* (pp. 111–131). Madison, CT: International Universities Press.

Volkan, V. D., & Ast, G. (2001). Curing Gitta's "leaking body": Actualized unconscious fantasies and therapeutic play. *Journal of Clinical Psychoanalysis, 10*: 567–606.

Volkan, V. D., Ast, G., & Greer, W. (2002). *Third Reich in the Unconscious*. New York: Routledge.

Wahlberg, K.-E., Wynne, L. C., Oja, H., Keskitalo, P., Pykäläinen, L., Lahti, I., Moring, J., Naarala , M., Sorri, A., Seitamaa, M., Läksy, K., Kolassa , J., & Tienari, P. (1997). Gene-environment interaction in vulnerability to schizophrenia: Findings from the Finnish Family Study of Schizophrenia. *American Journal of Psychiatry, 154*: 355–362.

Wang, A. W., Avramopoulos, D., Lori, A., Mulle, J., Conneely, K., Powers, A., Duncan, E., Almli, L., Massa, N., McGrath, J., Schwartz, A. C., Goes, F. S., Weng, L., Wang, R., Yolken, R., Ruczinski, I., Gillespie, C. F., Jovanovic, T., Ressler, K., Pulver, A. E., & Pearce, B. D. (2019). Genome-wide association study in two populations to determine genetic variants associated with Toxoplasma gondii infection and relationship to schizophrenia risk. *Progress in Neuro-Psychopharmacology & Biological Psychiatry, 92*: 133–147.

Wang, L.-Y., Chen, S.-F., Chiang, J.-H., Hsu, C.-Y., & Shen, Y.-C. (2018). Autoimmune diseases are associated with an increased risk of schizophrenia: A nationwide population-based cohort study. *Schizophrenia Research, 202*: 297–302.

Warman, D. M., & Beck, A. T. (2003). Cognitive behavioral therapy for schizophrenia: An overview of treatment. *Cognitive and Behavioral Practice, 10*: 248–254.

Watson, C. J., Thomas, R. H., Solomon, T., Michael, B. D., Nicholson, T. R., & Pollak, T. A. (2021). COVID-19 and psychosis risk: Real or delusional concern? *Neuroscience Letters, 741*: 135491.

Weigel, S., & Scharbert, G. (2016). *A Neuro-Psychoanalytical Dialogue for Bridging Freud and the Neurosciences*. New York: Springer.

Weininger, B. I. (1938). Psychotherapy during convalescence from psychosis. *Psychiatry: Journal for the Study of Interpersonal Processes, 2*: 257–264.

Weiser, M., Reichenberg, A., Rabinowitz, J., Kaplan, Z., Caspi, A., Yasvizky, R., Mark, M., Knobler, H. Y., Nahon, D., & Davidson, M. (2003). Self-reported drug abuse in male adolescents with behavioral disturbances, and follow-up for future schizophrenia. *Biological Psychiatry, 54*: 655–660.

Weisman, A. G., & López, S. R. (1997). An attributional analysis of emotional reactions to schizophrenia in Mexican and Anglo American cultures. *Journal of Applied Social Psychology, 27*: 223–244.

Werner, H., & Kaplan, B. (1984). *Symbol Formation*. Hillsdale, NJ: Psychology Press.

Whitaker, R. (2002). *Mad in America: Bad Science, Bad Medicine, and the Enduring Mistreatment of the Mentally Ill*. Cambridge, MA: Basic Books.

White, T., Cullen, K., Rohrer, L. M., Karatekin, C., Luciana, M., Schmidt, M., Hongwanishkul, D., Kumra, S., Schulz, S. C., & Lim, K. O. (2008). Limbic structures and networks in children and adolescents with schizophrenia. *Schizophrenia Bulletin, 34*: 18–29.

Will, O. (1964). Schizophrenia and the therapeutic field. *Contemporary Psychoanalysis, 34*: 89–97.

Williams, L. M., Das, P., Liddell, B. J., Olivieri, G., Peduto, A. S., David, A. S., Gordon, E., & Harris, A. W. F. (2007). Fronto-limbic and autonomic disjunctions to negative emotion distinguish schizophrenia subtypes. *Psychiatry Research: Neuroimaging, 155*: 29–44.

Willick, M. S. (2001). Psychoanalysis and schizophrenia: A cautionary tale. *Journal of the American Psychoanalytic Association, 49*: 27–56.

Winnicott, D. W. (1953). Transitional objects and transitional phenomena. A study of the first not-me possession. *International Journal of Psychoanalysis, 34*: 89–97.

Winnicott, D. W. (1971). *Playing and Reality*. Oxford: Penguin.

Winterer, G. (2006). Cortical microcircuits in schizophrenia—The dopamine hypothesis revisited. *Pharmacopsychiatry, 39*: S68–S71.

Włodarczyk, A., Szarmach, J., Cubała, W. J., & Wiglusz, M. S. (2017). Benzodiazepines in combination with antipsychotic drugs for schizophrenia: GABA-ergic targeted therapy. *Psychiatria Danubina, 29*: 345–348.

Wortinger, L. A., Engen, K., Barth, C., Lonning, V., Jørgensen, K. N., Andreassen, O. A., Haukvik, U. K., Vaskinn, A., Ueland, T., & Agartz, I. (2020). Obstetric complications and intelligence in patients on the schizophrenia-bipolar spectrum and healthy participants. *Psychological Medicine, 50*: 1914–1922.

Wotruba, D., Michels, L., Buechler, R., Metzler, S., Theodoridou, A., Gerstenberg, M., Walitza, S., Kollias, S., Rössler, W., & Heekeren, K. (2014). Aberrant coupling within and across the default mode, task-positive, and salience network in subjects at risk for psychosis. *Schizophrenia Bulletin, 40*: 1095–1104.

Xiao, J., Prandovszky, E., Kannan, G., Pletnikov, M. V., Dickerson, F., Severance, E. G., & Yolken, R. H. (2018). Toxoplasma gondii: Biological parameters of the connection to schizophrenia. *Schizophrenia Bulletin, 44*: 983–992.

Xu, J., He, G., Zhu, J., Zhou, X., St Clair, D., Wang, T., Xiang, Y., Zhao, Q., Xing, Q., Liu, Y., Wang, L., Li, Q., He, L., & Zhao, X. (2015). Prenatal nutritional deficiency reprogrammed postnatal gene expression in mammal brains: Implications for schizophrenia. *International Journal of Neuropsychopharmacology, 18*: 1–9.

Xu, L., Qi, X., Zhu, C., & Wan, L. (2018). Activation of IL-8 and its participation in cancer in schizophrenia patients: New evidence for the autoimmune hypothesis of schizophrenia. *Neuropsychiatric Disease and Treatment, 14*: 3393–3403.

Xu, X. J., & Jiang, G. S. (2015). Niacin-respondent subset of schizophrenia—a therapeutic review. *European Review for Medical and Pharmacological Sciences, 19*: 988–997.

Zandifar, A., & Badrfam, R. (2020). COVID-19: Considering the prevalence of schizophrenia in the coming decades. *Psychiatry Research, 288*: 112982.

Zarrei, M., MacDonald, J. R., Merico, D., & Scherer, S. W. (2015). A copy number variation map of the human genome. *Nature Reviews Genetics, 16*: 172–183.

Zhang, F., Gu, W., Hurles, M. E., & Lupski, J. R. (2009). Copy number variation in human health, disease, and evolution. *Annual Review of Genomics and Human Genetics, 10*: 451–481.

Zhenxing, Y., Longkun, L., & Miaoxin, L. (2018). De novo mutations as causes of schizophrenia. *Psychiatry Research, 270*: 1168–1169.

Zimmer-Bensch, G. (2018). Diverse facets of cortical interneuron migration regulation—Implications of neuronal activity and epigenetics. *Brain Research, 1700*: 160–169.

Zullino, D. F., Manghi, R., Rathelot, T., Khan, R., & Khazaal, Y. (2010). Cannabis causes schizophrenia? So does nicotine. *Addiction Research & Theory, 18*: 601–605.

Index

Abse, D. W., 125
abuse
    childhood, 1–17, 18–19
    physical, 17–18
    sexual, 16–19
    substance, 5, 9, 19, 26, 147
ACC *see* anterior cingulate cortex
Adam, M. A., 13, 114
Adams, D. D., 55
adolescence, 4, 19–20
adopted children, 71, 118
adult psychotic self, 88–89, 105–106,
        121–122, 130, 135–137
Agarwal, V., 55
Agbeli, M. O., 37
aggression, 32, 47, 73–74, 80, 85–86,
        88, 91, 99, 101, 160, 164
Akhtar, S., 88, 90
Alanen, Y. O., 76, 113
Albert, N., 38
alcohol(ism), 14–15, 20, 146–147
Allen, M., 135

Altshuler, D. M., 10, 11
Alvarez-Jimenez, M., 51
amafufunyana disorder, 157, 164–165
Angyal, A., 76
anterior cingulate cortex (ACC),
        31, 34, 69
acetylation, 13
acetylcysteine, 54
Applegate, J., 153
Apprey, M., 93
Arlow, J. A., 74
Arnaiz, A., 6
arousal, 41, 83–84
arthritis, 6, 27–28
Ashcroft, K., 18
Ashforth, A., 163
Ast, G., 95–96, 98
Ataque, 168–169
autoantibodies, 27–28
autoimmune, 23, 27–28, 53, 91
Ayurvedic, 55
Azrin, S. T., 61

bacteria, 22, 24, 28–29
Baker, A., 61
Bang, M., 54–55
Barkan, T., 32–33
Barrio, C., 151
Barrowclough, C., 58
basal ganglia, 30, 36, 49
Baumeister, A. A., 30, 50
Bayraktar, G., 13
Beck, A. T., 57
Bell, M., 152
Benderly, B., 79, 94
Beraki, S., 24
Berenbaum, H., 110
Berson, R. J., 168
Bhavsar, V., 150
Bhugra, D. 21, 150
biomarkers, 14–15, 55
Bioque, M., 29
bipolar, 12, 17, 32, 37
birth conditions, 20–21, 23, 154
Blokland, G., 12
Bonnigal-Katz, D., 110
Bosnak, R., 117
Boydell, J., 5
Boyer, B., 76, 84, 111, 140
Brahm, N. C., 53
Brakoulias, V., 48
Brambilla, P., 30
Braslow, J. T., 43
Bray, I., 5
Brazelton, M. T. B., 94
Brekke, J. S., 151
Brenner, C., 74
Bresnahan, M., 21
Brodmann's area 9, 32
Brown, A. S., 26, 62
Brown, S., 6
Bruscato, W., 152

Buckley, L., 55, 57
Buka, S. L., 26
Burckhardt, G., 47
Burnham, D. L., 76, 94
Burns, J., 40
Butler, P. D., 21
Byrn, M., 21
Burckhardt, G., 47

Cain, A. C., 96
Cain, B. S., 96
Calegari, F., 13
Cameron, N., 25, 122, 126
Cancro, R., 67
cannabis, 9, 19–20, 52, 62
cannibalism, 120, 131, 158–161
Capasso, R. M., 6
Capgras syndrome, 168
capsulotomy, 50
Cardiazol, 44
Carré, J. M., 165
Caruso, J. P., 48
Cary, B., 158
casein, 28
Caseras, X., 11
Casey, D. E., 6
Castiglione, J., 28
Castle, D. J., 4
castration, 162 *see also vagina dentata*
    anxiety, 84–85, 162
    auto-, 99
Cattane, N., 15, 29
CBT *see* cognitive behavioral therapy
cerebral blood flow, 54
Çetingök, M., 146
Chan, S. K. W., 6, 61,
Chant, D., 21
Chaudhry, I. D., 53
Chaudhuri, T. K., 54

Cheng, Y., 68
Cheniaux, E., 4
child(hood)
    abuse, 16–19
    adopted, 71
    attachment, 69
    cognitive impairment in, 38
    development, 133–135
    early, 111
    MRI image, 70
    and parents, 75, 90–91, 93–101,
        126, 138
    rearing, 153–156
    schizophrenia, 34
    trauma, 42, 114
    viral infections in, 24
Chiu, V. W., 58
chlorpromazine, 48, 55
cholinergic transmission, 31
chromatin, 13
Chua, T. H., 6
Chused, J. F., 126
Chwastiak, L. A., 6
Clair, D. S., 11
CNV see copy number variation
cognitive abnormalities, 4, 25, 29,
        31–32, 37–39, 41, 50, 84
cognitive behavioral therapy (CBT),
        57–59, 61, 64, 82
cognitive symptoms, 36, 49–50,
        52, 63
Colangeli, R., 92, 114
Colonna, A. B., 95
Consoli, A. J., 168
Conus, P., 52, 115
copy number variation (CNV), 10–11
coronaviruses, 23–24, 173
cortex/cortical, 10–11, 26, 31–32,
        34–35, 41, 46, 49, 56, 69, 83

corticogenesis, 11
corticosteroids, 28
corticostriatal, 32
Cotton, H., 22–23
countertransference, 69, 76, 122,
        127, 136, 142 see also
        transference
Cowan, H. R., 25
COVID-19, 24–25, 173
C-reactive protein (CRP), 54
Cree, 158
CRP see C-reactive protein
Cullen, A. E., 27–28
cultural elements, xvi, 5, 117, 135,
        146, 150, 152, 155–157,
        159, 163–165, 168–169,
        171–173
Cumming, P., 31
cytokine, 11, 26–27, 53–54
cytomegalovirus, 23–24
cytosine, 13

DAAO see D-amino acid oxidase
Dalman, C., 24
D-amino acid oxidase (DAAO), 53
D'Astous, M., 50
Davenport, S., 111
Davis, J. M., 51
davunetide, 54
DBS see deep brain stimulation
De Luca, V., 33
De Masi, F., 111
Dean, B., 32–33, 50
Dean, K., 8, 30
deep brain stimulation (DBS), 36,
        48–50, 63
Dellario, D., 4
delusion, 4, 16, 18–19, 41, 73, 88,
        94, 98–99, 104, 115, 141,

145–147, 150, 160–162,
168–169
delusional, 3–4, 58, 97, 127, 158,
166, 169
dementia, 25, 37
demon, 14, 16, 152
dendritic spines, 32
developed and developing nations, 6,
21, 147
depositing, 96–97
depression or depressive, 5, 12, 18,
46–47, 57–58, 86, 98, 130,
161, 173
Devinsky, O., 150
Dhat, 168–169
Dickson, H., 38
Dion, G. L., 4
Divac, N., 51
DNA, 13–15, 91–92
DNA methyltransferase inhibitors
(DNMT), 15
Doody, G. A., 5
dopamine, 14, 30–31, 35–36, 38,
50–53, 56, 63
dopamine D receptor gene
(DRD), 35
dopaminergic, 19, 30–31, 35–36,
69, 151
Dorpat, T. L., 79
dorsolateral prefrontal cortex, 26, 31
dosReis, S., 51
doughnut personality, 85–86, 88,
96, 105
Downing, D. L., 76, 110
DRD see dopamine D receptor gene
Duggal, H. S., 99
Dully, H., 48
Dykxhoorn, J., 20
dysbiosis, 29

Eberhard, J., 8
ECT see electroshock
Edwards, F. S., 164–165
Eecke, W., 111
ego, 72–80, 83–85, 90–91, 95–97,
99–102, 105, 111, 115,
119–121, 126, 131, 133,
137, 141
Ekstein, R., 126
electroacupuncture, 55
electroshock (ECT), 44–47, 55
Ellenbroek, B., 11
Elwin, V., 166
embodied dreamwork, 117
Emde, R. E., 80, 153
encapsulation, 102–103, 105–106
endotoxins, 29
Enger, C., 7
Ensink, K., 165
environmental factors, 15, 29, 54,
91, 153
epigenetics, 12–15, 28, 91–92, 114
epinephrine, 52
Erikson, E. H., 130
evolution, 40, 73–74, 79, 95, 104, 125,
133, 135
Ewing, J. A., 125
Eyles, D. W., 12

Fairbairn, W. R. D., 110
Fakr, E., 41
Fan, J. B., 33
Fatemi, S. H., 26
Fearon, P., 21, 151
Fenichel, O., 73–74, 84
Ferenczi, S., 109
Fiamberti, A., 47
Fierini, A., 24–25
Findlay, I. J., 6

Fisch, R. Z., 167
Fischmann, T., 91
Fleck, S., 75
Flegr, J., 24
Fleming, C., 48
fMRI *see* functional magnetic
    resonance imaging
focal sepsis, 22–23
Fonseca, L., 24
Forman, M., 48
Fornito, A., 34
Fors, B. M., 6
Foussias, G., 52
Francis, J. L., 30, 50
Frankle, W. G., 33
Frantzis, B. K., 163
Freeman, W., 47–48
Freud, A., 75
Freud S., 67–68, 72–75, 90,
    109–110
Fröhlich, F., 47
Fromm-Reichmann, F., 75, 94, 109
fronto-temporal dysconnectivity
    hypotheses, 35
Fu, S., 38
Fuchs, S. H., 120
Fujita, K., 153
functional magnetic resonance
    imaging (fMRI), 35, 68,
    71 *see also* magnetic
    resonance imaging
Furer, M., 83, 133
Furnham, A., 148

gamma-aminobutyric acid (GABA),
    14, 31–32
Garfield, D., 76
Garver, D., 5
Gault, J., 36, 49–50

Gazdag, G., 46
Gearon, J. S., 19
gene(s), 8, 10–15, 24, 27, 31, 33, 35,
    38, 40, 91
genetics, 8–13, 20, 28, 32, 40, 71,
    91–92, 114–115, 142, 156
Gibbs, P. L., 76, 91, 110
Gibson, E. L., 151
Gil, A., 17
Gilmore, J. H., 8
Gilmour, G., 32
Giovacchini, P., 76, 126
Girdler, S. J., 56
Glass, J., 84
glutamate, 31–32, 52
GMB *see* human gut microbiota
Gold, C., 58
Gomes, F. V., 20
Gong, H., 13, 114
González de Chávez, M., 43
Gonzalez-Flores, B. L., 60
Gorman, J.M., 92
Gössler, R., 99
Gottdiener, W. H., 111
Gottlieb, J., 165
Grace, A. A., 20
Gray, L., 32
Green, M., 79, 96, 120
Greenacre, P., 95
Greenspan, S., 79, 94
Grignon, S., 5
Grotstein, J. S., 76, 85, 111
Gründer, G., 31
Guadalupe, L. A. O., 163
Gulsuner, S., 10, 11
Gur, R. E., 40
Gürel, Ç., 13, 15
gut, 28–29, 63
Gyuris, J., 99

Hadar, R., 49
Hagen, C. A., 161
Hagiwara, H., 50
Hallowell, A. I., 161
hallucinations, 1–3, 16–19, 47, 59, 87, 96, 115
Hartmann, H., 73–74
Harwell, C. C., 13, 114
Hashimoto, T., 31
HDAC *see* histone deacetylase inhibitors
Healy, D., 6
Heckel, T., 11
Hendrick, I, 22
Heng, H. H., 11
Henssler, J., 21
heritability, 9–11
Hernandez, E. I., 46–47
herpes simplex virus (HSV), 23, 26
Hilker, R., 10
hippocampus, 10, 35–36, 56
Hiraoka, A., 163
histone, 13–15, 91
histone deacetylase inhibitors (HDAC), 15
histone demethylase inhibitors (HMT), 15
Hitler, A., 123
HMT *see* histone demethylase inhibitors
Hodge, J. M., 23
Hoeffding, L. K., 28
Hoffmann, K., 55
Hong, J., 54–55
Holocaust, 21, 97, 155
Høyersten, J. G., 43
HSV *see* herpes simplex virus
Hu, P. C., 163
Hua, M., 35

Huang, T., 11
Huguelet, P., 61
human gut microbiota (GMB), 29
Hutchinson, g., 150
Hwang, J. Y., 13, 114
Hwang, W. C., 162–163
Hwang, W.-C., 151
hydrogen peroxide, 53
hydrotherapy, 43
hydroxytryptamine, 52
hypofrontality, 32

Iannitelli, A., 114
immigration, 9, 20–21, 28, 44, 62, 135, 150
infantile non-psychotic self, 100
infantile psychotic self, 100–102, 165
infections, 9, 22, 25, 62
infectious agents, 22–23, 26–27, 91
inflammation, 11, 25–26, 28–29, 53–54, 63
insula, 69
insulin, 44
interferon, 54
İpçi, K., 60
internalization–externalization cycle, 80–81, 96, 116, 118, 121–123, 125, 127, 129, 141

Jacobson, E., 75, 78
Janssen, I., 16
Jauhur, S., 58
Jentsch, J. D., 32
Jia, J., 55
Jiang, G. S., 56
Jobe, E. M., 13
Joffe, W. G., 84
Johnson, B., 69, 115
Jones, E., 26

Joukamaa, M., 6
Joyal, C. C., 19
Juckel, G., 55
Jung, C. G., 109

Kane, J. M., 51
Kapelski, P., 33
Kaplan, B., 118, 134
Kapsambelis, V., 111
Kastrup, M. C., 151
Kelly, D. L., 181
Kelly, K., 100
Kernberg, O., 78–80, 126, 133
Keshavan, M., 10
Kessler, R. J., 68
Khandaker, G. M., 24
Kim, H., 18
Kippin, T., 32
Kitcher, P., xiii–xiv
Klein, G., xiii
Klein, M., 76, 122
Kline, J., 111
Knight, J., 27, 53
Koch, E., 38
Kohler, C. G., 41
Kohut, H., 79
Koro, 168–169
Kortegaard, H. M., 111
Kosugi, D., 153
Kozloff, N., 24
Kraguljac, N. V., 51
Kreutz, M. R., 13
Krippner, S., 166
Krogmann, A.,52, 55
Kroll, J. L., 5
Kuba, R., 24
Kuijpers, H., 163
Kumar, V., 31
Kurihara, T. 149

Lacan, J., 111
Lachmann, A., 149
Lai, G., 150
Lamster, F., 58
Landes, R., 161
Landy, D., 160
Lanktree, M. B., 11
Laskemoen, J. F., 39
Laursen, T. M., 6
Lawrence, R., 58
Leão, T. S., 21, 151
Lee, K. W., 10–11
Lee, Y., 163
Lehtinen, V., 52
Lehtonen, J, 71, 80
Leonhardt, B. L., 18
Lester, D., 7
Leucht, S., 6, 51
leucotomy, 47
Leuzinger-Bohleber, M., 91
Levin, F.M., 115
Lewis, S., 51
Lewis-Fernáandez, R., 168
Lidz, T., 75
Lieberman, F., 154
Lieberman, J. A., 51–52
life expectancy, 6
Lim, R., 163
Lima, A., 47
limbic system, 34, 40, 151
Lin, K.-M., 163
Lindberg, J., 159
lobotomy, 45, 47–48
Loewald, H., 126
LoF see loss of function
London, N., 72, 73
López, S. R., 149
López-Muñoz, F., 48
Lorenzo, C.V., 32

loss of function (LoF), 11
Lublin, H., 8
Lucas, R., 111
Luhrmann, T. M., 151
lupus erythematosus, 27
Lustenberger, C., 47
Lysaker, P., 17

Mackler, D., 76
magnetic resonance imaging (MRI), 70–71 see also functional magnetic resonance imaging
magnetic resonance spectroscopy, 31
Mahler, M., 76, 83, 133
major depressive disorder (MDD), 46
major histocompatibility complex (MHC), 10–11
Marini, S., 71, 115
Marneros, A., 4
Masciotra, L., 31
Mateen, B. A., 13
Maurel, M., 39
Mausbach, B. T., 151
May, P., 110, 168
McCarroll, S. A., 10–11
McClellan, J. M., 10, 11
McDougall, J., 94
McGee, H., 160
McGrath, J. J., 5, 62
McQueeney, D. A., 57
MDD see major depressive disorder
medication, 3, 5–6, 11, 15, 26, 32–33, 35, 37–39, 49–52, 54, 57–58, 60–64, 86–87, 110, 113–114, 116–117, 163–164
megalomania, 22, 72, 86, 88, 96, 105
Menninger, K., 22, 25
MERS see Middle East respiratory syndrome

mesenchymal stem cells, 54
mesolimbic, 31, 151
messenger RNA, 13
metapsychology, 31, 65, 67–68, 71, 74, 76, 88, 82, 114, 151
methylation, 13–15, 91
methylcytosine, 13
methyltransferase, 15
Metrazol, 44
Meyer, U., 15
MHC see major histocompatibility complex
Middle East respiratory syndrome (MERS), 25
minocycline, 54
miR-137, 10
Miller, B. J., 54
Miller, C. A., 13
Miller, M. J., 156
Miller, P., 19
Mills, J., 78, 110
miRNAs see non-coding micro RNAs
Mishra, A., 55
Mitsadali, I., 56
Mittal, V. A., 57,
Modell, A.H., 68
molecular scars, 15
Møllerhøj, J., 61
Moniz, E., 47
Moore, L. D., 13
Moran, E. K., 37
morbidity, 5, 22, 37
Moreno, J. L., 26
Morgan, V., 4
Mosri, D. F., 69, 115
mothering
    borderline or psychotic, 94
    unconscious fantasies, 93–94
    schizophrenogenic, 94

Mother Theresa, 88
mourning, 141
MRI *see* magnetic resonance
      imaging
mRNA *see* messenger RNA
Mulder, M. B., 148
Mulle, J. G., 9
Mullen, P. E., 17
Mueser, K. T., 110
Murray, R. M., 19, 26

Nelson, C. L. M., 38
neocortex, 150
Nervios, 168–169
neuromodulation, 44, 46–47, 49, 63,
      171–172
Newman, L. M., 95
new object, 126, 141
Ng, B.-Y., 163
niacin, 56
Niebuhr, D. W., 24
Nightingale, L.C., 57
Nixon, N. L., 5
N-methyl-D-aspartate (NMDA),
      31–32, 52
NNAI *see* non-neurological
      autoimmune disorders
Noack, F., 13
non-coding micro RNAs
      (miRNAs), 13
non-neurological autoimmune
      (NNAI) disorders, 28
non-psychotic disorders, 17, 18
non-psychotic self, 105
non-steroidal anti-inflammatory
      drugs (NSAIDS), 54
Novick, J., 100
NSAIDS *see* non-steroidal anti-
      inflammatory drugs

nucleus accumbens, 49
Nyffeler, M., 26

object relations, xv–xiii, 9, 39, 69,
      77–82, 84, 87, 98, 110, 112,
      121–122, 134, 142 *see also*
      new object
obsessive-compulsive disorder
      (OCD), 49–50, 63
obstetric complications, 21
Ødegård, Ø., 150
Ohara, K., 31, 56
Olinick, S. L., 116
Omega-3 fatty acids, 54, 56
Opler, M. K., 146, 157
orbitofrontal cortex , 83
organismic panic, 83–84, 86–87,
      89–90, 105–106, 116,
      119, 129–131, 135, 137–138
Ottet, M.-C., 35

pandemic, 22, 24–25, 173
Pandurangi, A. K., 55
Pang, N., 55
Pankow, G., 110
Pao, P-.N., 73, 76, 83–84
paranoia, 41, 145–147, 159, 161
Pardiñas, A., 11
Parle, J., 165
pars reticulata, 49
pathogenesis, 12, 28, 35, 51, 71, 95,
      111, 138
Patterson, P. H., 62
PDE10A *see* phosphodiesterase
      10A enzyme
Peltzer, K., 21, 165
pemphigoid, 28
penis, 98–99, 131
Pettit, T., 57

Phii Pob, 168
phosphodiesterase 10A enzyme
(PDE10A), 52
phosphorylation, 13
Piblokto, 160
Potvin, S., 23
Poulet, E., 47
Prandovszky, E., 28
Prasad, K. M. R., 26
Pratt, L.A., 6
prefrontal, 26, 30–31, 41, 47, 49, 56
Presley, E., 97
prevalence, 4–5, 7, 21, 23
psychosurgery, xiii, 47–48, 63, 171
psychotherapy, xiv–xvii, 5, 9, 15, 18,
57, 61, 64, 68–70, 78, 82,
106, 110, 113–114, 116,
120, 172
cognitive-behavioral, 57–59, 61,
64, 82
group, 57
supportive, xv, 57, 119
psychotic personality organization, 103
Ptak, S. E., 149
Purhonen, M., 71
pyramidal, 31–32

qigong psychosis, 157, 162–163, 169

Rado, J., 46–47
Rakitzi, S., 61
Ramamourty, P., 168
Ran, M.-S., 7
Rapaport, D., 126
Rashno, M. M., 23
Rathbone, J., 55
reaching up, 84–85, 124, 162
Read, J., 16
regression in the service of the
other, 116

religiosity, 135, 150
Remington, G., 52
replacement children, 96–97
resting state effective connectivity
(rsEC), 35
Restrepo, D., 60–61
Richard, M. D., 53
Richetto, J., 15
rheumatoid arthritis, 6, 27–28
right-temporo-parietal junction
(TPJ), 69
RNA, 10, 13, 91
Robertson, B., 165
Robinson, D. S., 6
Roffman, J. L., 68
Rogers, J. P., 25
Rohrl, V. J., 160
Rokita, K., 18
Rosenbaum, B., 149
Rosenfeld, D., 102
Rosenfeld, H., 102
Roser, P., 19
Ross, C. A., 5
Roth, R. H., 32
rsEC *see* resting state effective
connectivity
Rumbaugh, G., 13
Ryan, J. E., 20

Sabe, M., 56
Saha, S., 6, 21
Salone, A., 115
Sanderson, I. T., 160
Sandler, J., 84
Saora disorder, 157–158, 164–167
Saravanan, B., 145, 148, 151
Sarter, M., 31
Saxe, R., 70–71
Scharbert, G., 114
schizoaffective disorder, 3–4, 18, 26

schizophreniform disorder, 3–4, 103, 163
schizophrenogenic, 23, 75, 94
schizotypal, 3, 17, 27, 103, 109
Schokking, I. D., 161
Schore, A. N., 83–84
Schulmann, G., 113, 122
Schulz, C., 76
Schürhoff, F., 17
Schwab, S. G., 8
Scull, A., 22–23
Searles, H., 76, 110, 116, 118
Seeman, P., 50
Segal, H., 122
selective regression, 73–74
Sells, J., 163
Sepehry, A. A., 33
serotonin, 14, 32–33, 52
Setién-Suero, E., 20
Severance, E. G., 27–29
shaman(s), 166–167
Shao, X., 11
Sheehan, J. P., 48
Shekunov, J., 21
Shimada, T., 56
Shonin, E., 58
Silva, M. A., 60–61
Sim, K., 6
Simeone, J. C., 5
Simpson, M. A., 151
Singh, B., 54
single nucleotide polymorphisms (SNPs), 11–12
Sklar, P., 33
Smigielski, L., 14, 114
SNPs see single nucleotide polymorphisms
social defeat, 151
Solnit, A. J., 96
Sommer, I. E., 55

Spanos, N. P., 165
Spataro, J., 17
Spitz, R., 86
Staudt, M., 47
Steel, C., 59
Stefansson, H., 11
Stern, D. N., 153
Stone, L., 75
Stone, M. H., 110
stressors, 25, 54, 62, 163–164, 166, 169, 173
subcortical ergotropic arousal, 83
substantia nigra, 49
Sudak, D. M., 57
suicide, 7, 24, 94, 104, 146
suitable targets, 134
Sullivan, H. S., 75
Sullivan, P., 10
Sumiyoshi, T., 33
superego, 74, 79–80, 90, 97, 126, 140–141
superior frontal gyrus, 69
surgery, 22–23, 50, 63, 94, 98, 103
Susto, 168–169
Sutterland, A. L., 24
Suvisaari, J. M., 5
Suwanlert, S., 168
Szumlinski, K. K., 32

TAAR see trace amine-associated receptor
Tähkä, V., 90, 126
Tandon, R., 51
Tansella, M., 30
Taquet, M., 24
tardive dyskinesia, 49–50, 86
Tek, C., 6
teratogen, 27
THC, 54
Thomann, P. A., 46

Thorazine *see* chlorpromazine
Thygesen, J. H., 11
Tidd, C., 109
Tienari, P., 71
TMS *see* transcranial magnetic stimulation
Tochigi, M., 21
Torrey, E. F., 9, 24
Torsti, M., 94,
Toxoplasma gondii (T. gondii), 9, 23–24, 28, 62
Toxoplasmosis *see* Toxoplasma gondii
TPJ *see* right-temporo-parietal junction
trace amine-associated receptor (TAAR), 52
transcranial magnetic stimulation (TMS), 47
transference, xvii, 69, 75, 81, 90, 96, 110, 119, 122, 125–127, 138, 140 *see also* countertransference
transitional object, 95–96, 142
trophotropic arousal, 83
Tropp, J., 164
Trottier, M., 5
Trudeau, K. J., 6
Tsapakis, E.-M., 19
Turkington, D., 57
Tustin, F., 102
twin(s), 9, 71, 95

Udina, M., 168
ukuthwasa, 164
Ungvari, G. S., 46

vaccine, 55
vagina dentata, 147

Valon, P., 110
valproic acid, 15
Varvin, S., 147
Vaucher, J., 20
ventral cortex, 49
ventral striatum, 49
ventral tegmental area, 36, 50
Verlingue, M., 168–169
Vidal, S., 61
viruses, 23–24
Vitebsky, P., 116
Vogel, M., 17
Volavka, J., 147
Volkan, K., 16, 43, 45, 95, 97–98, 104, 117, 142, 168
Volkan, V. D., 44, 76, 80, 84, 88, 90, 95–100, 102–104, 106, 111, 116, 118–120, 123, 125–126, 128, 130–131, 133–135, 138, 142, 155–156

Wahlberg, K.-E., 71
Wang, A. W., 24
Wang, L.-Y., 27
Warman, D. M., 57
Watson, C., 24–25
Watts, J., 47
Weigel, S., 114
Weigert, E., 75
Weininger, B., 109
Weiser, M., 19
Weisman, A. G., 149
Welham, J. L., 21
wendigo psychosis, 157–158, 161, 164–167
Werner, H., 118, 134
Whitaker, R., 43–44
White, T., 35, 149
Wildenauer, D. B., 8

Will, O., 76
Wilkes, K. V., xiii–xiv
Williams, L. M., 41
Willick, M. S., 114
Winnicott, D. W., 94–95, 153
Winterer, G., 3
Włodarczyk, A., 32
Wong, L., 148
world destruction fantasy, 73
Wortinger, L. A., 21
Wotruba, D., 35

Xiao, J., 24
Xu, J., 56

Xu, L., 27
Xu, X. J., 13, 56, 114

Yolken, R. H., 28–29, 63
Youn, J., 11

Zandifar, A., 24
Zhao, X., 13
Zarrei, M., 10
Zellner, M., 68
Zhang, F., 11
Zhenxing, Y. 11
Zimmer-Bensch, G., 13
Zullino, D. F., 19